The Authorities

Powerful Wisdom from Leaders in the Field

YVONNE ABOU-NADER
Retired Cancer Survivor

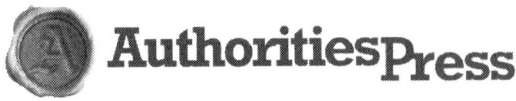

Publisher
Authorities Press
Markham, ON
Canada

Printed in the United States and the United Kingdom.

FOREWORD

Experts are to be admired for their knowledge, but they often remain unrecognized by the general public because they save their information and insights for paying customers and clients. There are many experts in a given field, but their impact is limited to the handful of people with whom they work.

Unlike experts, authorities share their knowledge and expertise far more broadly, so they make a big impact on the world. Authorities become known and admired as leading experts and, as such, typically do very well economically and professionally. Most authorities are also mature enough to know that part of the joy of monetary success is the accompanying moral and spiritual obligation to give back.

Many people want to learn and work with well-respected and generous authorities, but don't always know where to find them. They may be known to their peers, or within a specific community, but have not had the opportunity to reach a wider audience. At one time, they might have submitted a proposal to the For Dummies or Chicken Soup for the Soul series of books, but it's now almost impossible to get accepted as a new author in such branded book series.

It is more than fitting that Raymond Aaron, an internationally known and respected authority in his own right, would be the one to recognize the need for a new venue in which authorities could share their considerable knowledge with readers everywhere. As the only author ever to be included in both of the book series mentioned above, Raymond has had the opportunity to give back and he understands how crucial it is for authorities to have a platform from which to share their expertise.

I have known and worked with Raymond for a number of years and consider him a valued friend and talented coach. He knows how to spot talented and knowledgeable people and he desires to see them prosper. Over the years, success coaching and speaking engagements around the world have made it possible for Raymond to meet many of these talented authorities. He recognizes and relates to their passion and enthusiasm for what they do, as well as their desire to share what they know. He tells me that's why he created this new nonfiction branded book series, The Authorities.

Dr. Nido Qubein
President, High Point University

TABLE OF CONTENTS

INTRODUCTION

This book introduces you to *The Authorities* — individuals who have distinguished themselves in life and in business. Authorities make a big impact on the world. Authorities are leaders in their chosen fields. Authorities typically do very well financially, and are evolved enough to know that part of the joy of monetary success is the accompanying social, moral and spiritual obligation to give back.

Authorities are not just outstanding. They are also *known* to be outstanding.

This additional element begins to explain the difference between two strategic business and life concepts — one that seems great, but isn't, and the other that fills in the essential missing gap of the first.

The first concept is "the expert."

What is an expert? The real definition is …

EXPERT: *a person who knows stuff*

People who have attained a very senior academic degree (like a PhD or an MD) definitely know stuff. People who read voraciously and retain what they read definitely know stuff. Unfortunately, just because you know stuff does not mean that anyone respects the fact that you do. Even though some experts are successful, alas, most are not — because knowing stuff is not enough.

Well, then, what is the missing piece?

What the expert lacks, "the authority" has. The authority both knows stuff and is *known* to know stuff. So, more simply …

AUTHORITY: *a person who is known as an expert*

The difference is not subtle. The difference is not merely semantic. The difference is enormous.

When it comes to this subject, there are actually three categories in which people fall:

- People who don't know much and are unsuccessful in life and in business. Most people fall in this category.

- People who know stuff, but still don't leave much of a footprint in the world. There are a lot of people like this.

- Experts who are also *known* as experts become authorities and authorities are always wondrously successful. Authorities are able to contribute more to humanity through both their chosen work and their giving back.

This book is about the highest category, *The Authorities* — people who have reached the peak in their field and are known as such.

You will definitely know some of The Authorities in this book, especially since there are some world-famous ones. Others are just as exceptional, but you may not yet know about them. Our featured author, for example, is Yvonne Abou-Nader. Yvonne has always felt a calling to care for others. As a nurse, her career centered around general intensive care and cardiothoracic nursing. She loved her patients and enjoyed caring for them but retired at the age of 73 after she was diagnosed with breast cancer. Learning firsthand how difficult a cancer diagnosis can be, Yvonne is inspired to share what she learned so that she may help others.

You must read her chapter, "Coping with Cancer," where she shares her firsthand experiences being diagnosed with cancer, undergoing treatment, and going through recovery. With her guidance, you will be inspired to face cancer or any other obstacle that comes your way with a positive attitude and determination to overcome. Yvonne shares her research so that you can make informed decisions on treatment, should you ever need it. With her personal experience and knowledge of cancer treatments, planning a course of treatment will be much less daunting.

Read each chapter carefully to learn and to see the business potential that may be possible between yourself and each one of *The Authorities*. You may well be able to become their client or, possibly, do business with them in other ways.

They are *The Authorities*. Learn from them. Connect with them. Let them uplift you. Learning from them and working with them is the secret ingredient for success which may well allow you to rise to the level of Authority soon.

To be considered for inclusion in a subsequent edition of *The Authorities*, register to attend a future event at www.aaron.com/events where you will be interviewed and considered.

Coping With Cancer

YVONNE ABOU-NADER

I vividly remember the morning of April 7, 2013. I had recently moved from London and was looking to buy a house in Chelmsford to be near my sister and her family. That morning, I was drying myself after a shower when I noticed a red groove underneath my left breast. An alarm bell rang in my head as I stared at the groove. I just knew, in that moment, that I had cancer. Until then, I never noticed the groove. I was not in the habit of examining myself because I never dreamed that cancer would happen to me. I stared at the red, grooved patch and my fears ran wild as I imagined the worst.

I lived with it for ten days while waiting for an appointment with my general practitioner. I was a mess during those ten days! Confused and anxious, I was not sleeping well and could not concentrate on my work. I continuously wondered how this could have happened to me. Suddenly, the importance of conducting self-exams to feel for lumps became all too real. My last mammogram had been four years ago; I should have had one two years prior, but somehow neglected to have it done.

I strongly encourage women over the age of thirty to examine their breasts and feel for lumps. If a lump is detected, diagnosis and treatment will begin early and there will be a better chance of eradicating the cancer and preventing it from spreading to other organs, increasing the survival rate.

I kept my discovery to myself because I did not want my family to worry about me. While waiting for my appointment, I went to Chicago for my cousin's funeral. Throughout the service, I kept thinking that my turn would be next. I was terrified! Each time I undressed, the alarming red grooved patch on my breast jumped out at me. Fearing that something that looked this bad would surely be the nasty type of cancer with a low survival rate, I worried that it would be too late for successful treatment and that I would only survive a few months. Again, I kept my fears to myself and did not tell anyone.

After returning to the United Kingdom, it was time for my appointment with my general practitioner. He referred me to an oncologist who did a biopsy and scan. Two weeks later, I went back for the results of the biopsy and scan. Sitting in the waiting room, it felt like an eternity before my name was called. As time slowly passed, my mind raced with thoughts that made me even more anxious and nervous. Eventually, my name was called and I followed the nurse to the consultation room.

The oncology consultant stood up to shake my hand, indicated my chair, then waited for me to sit down. I asked him what the verdict was. He said that although he had the results of my preliminary biopsy and scan, he would need to conduct further tests. He told me that, unfortunately, he did not have good news; I had stage 3-4 breast cancer involving the lymph glands. I would need surgery before they would know the extent of my cancer.

This hit me like a ton of bricks! You can imagine how a person would react to such terrible news. The words "you have cancer" feel like a death sentence. In that moment, my world collapsed around me. Confused, shocked, angry, and scared, I repeated, "No...why me? What is happening? Why?" My first reaction was denial, even though I had heard the words I had feared all along.

HOW COULD THIS HAPPEN TO ME?

I sat there in shock and denial. What caused this? How could it happen to me? I eat the right foods and do not indulge in junk food, sugar cakes, or fizzy drinks. I do not smoke and only drink alcohol occasionally, such as one glass of wine when I go out for dinner. I exercise and work 12 hours a day, while feeling fit and well.

Upon telling me the news, the consultant realized that I was in a state of shock and asked the nurse to stay with me. She took me to a room and sat there with me, allowing me to talk and recover from the shock. I kept on repeating "Why, why?"

What had I done wrong to deserve this? What would happen to the elderly ladies who I look after and the other charitable work I do? The nurse patiently sat and listened to me vent my worries and react to the horrible news.

Once I gathered my wits, she gave me a leaflet and explained that I could get help from Macmillan nurses who specialize in cancer care in hospitals and in the community. She told me there was a telephone number if I wanted to talk to someone.

Macmillan Cancer Support is a program in the UK that offers support to people diagnosed with cancer. They understand that cancer affects every aspect of your life and work with you to help you as you deal with cancer. They can be there during treatments, they can help with job and money worries, they will listen if you just need to vent, help with benefit applications, and even offer emotional support to your whole family.

(For more info, visit www.macmillan.org.uk. It is a wonderful resource!)

On the way home from my consultation, I fixated on finding out what could be the cause of my cancer. It had not sunk in that my general practitioner had told me to stop the hormone replacement therapy (HRT). I had done this for ten years to relieve the symptoms of menopause. I eventually did stop the hormone treatments. The other contributory cause was stress, which can be an underlying cause of many diseases and illnesses. My stress level over the previous five years was enormous!

I spent the next three days on my own, not saying a word to my family or friends. Instead, I bottled up my emotions and reflected on what I could do and what action I would take. I knew I had to deal with the problem and face reality. However, I struggled to think clearly or concentrate as my mind raced with fears and worries.

On the fourth day, I called my sister and asked her to come for a visit. When she arrived, I broke the news to her and we both burst into tears. She then phoned my brother to tell him the sad news. I spoke with him and he gave me his support.

After sharing my news and allowing others to strengthen and sustain me, I was in a better place emotionally. I knew I must be positive and do the right thing to overcome the anxiety and stress so that my body could fight the cancer. I made up my mind that cancer was not going to kill me, and I would beat it no matter what it took.

WAITING FOR SURGERY

Waiting is so hard! I felt like I had to do something while waiting for my surgery, so I searched online for alternative cancer treatments in different countries. I was particularly intrigued with how cancer is treated in Japan and China. I recalled seeing a program on television about a clinic in China that treated people with cancer using natural herbs. This had also been done in Mexico with good results. I discussed these treatments with my sister and brother, along with my niece, who is a doctor. All three did not want me to go this route with my treatment.

So, I continued to wait. The ten weeks I had to wait for my surgery felt like ten years! It was an anxious and stressful time. I imagined the cancer spreading further throughout my body while I waited. I feared my prognosis would become worse with each passing day.

I carried on with my daily routine and tried to remain positive. I went to the theatre, concerts, seminars, and workshops to keep my mind occupied. I also spent time talking with friends who were always supportive and sympathetic. I continued to work three days a week so that I could be around people rather than staying home and focusing on my cancer.

Finally, it was time for my surgery. I was nervous, of course, but also strangely excited because I was going to have this invader removed from my body. When I awoke from surgery, the surgeon assured me that he removed the breast along with 14 lymph glands from under my left arm. Two of the lymph glands were large and malignant; the rest were small and nonmalignant but were sent for further tests.

After three days, I was discharged from the hospital with a drainage bag in my side, which drained excess fluid, mainly from the lymphatic system. Once I felt well enough to leave the house, I carried the drainage bag in a concealed carrier bag. I was renovating my house during this time, so I went around to the shops and bought supplies for the people working on my house. I kept myself busy so that I did not think about my situation. Then I was notified of an appointment to see the consultant to start chemotherapy.

CHEMOTHERAPY AND RADIOTHERAPY

I was told that I needed six treatments at three-week intervals, then six weeks after the chemo I would need 16 sessions of radiotherapy. I completed all the therapies, but I regret them to this day. In hindsight, I wish I had followed my gut feeling to have the surgery only. The side effects of chemotherapy and radiotherapy are not worth having them done, in my opinion. Although I do not know where I would be today if I had not had them, I would not have done these treatments had I known then what I know now.

Chemo and radiation are akin to poisoning your system. They lower your immunity, killing good cells as well as the cancer cells, and some of the side effects are irreversible. I experienced all the side effects from chemo, including losing all body hair, losing my fingernails and toenails, nausea, vomiting, loss of appetite, metallic taste (even water tasted metallic), weakness, insomnia, a burning sensation, and pain and burning on the soles of my feet. I also experienced memory loss; I knew what I wanted to say, but it would take me a couple of minutes to remember how to say it.

Additionally, I had a chest infection and neutropenic attack that required admission to the hospital for four days. My white blood cell count went down to zero! I was given antibiotics and upon discharge from the hospital, I took Vitamin B and Vitamin C supplements. I am partial to Vitamin C for building my immunity and keeping me clear of colds during the winter. I also ate nourishing fresh soup I cooked myself.

By the third week post-chemo treatment, I began to feel better. The following week I had another chemo treatment and the side effects began all over again. I ended up having only five chemotherapy sessions rather than the recommended six sessions.

FATEFUL CRUISE

Six weeks post-chemo it was time to begin radiotherapy. This took place in a different hospital which was a forty-five-minute commute from my home. My sister took me to all my radiotherapy appointments and kept me company during the treatment. The radiation burned my skin and left a lesion on my body. The side effects continue today. I suffer from a weak heart and weakened muscles.

I finished the course on the twenty-second of December and on the fourth of January I went on a cruise! I took a supply of wound dressings and anti-septic to dress the wound. I needed to get away; away from doctors and hospitals and treatments!

I flew to Miami where I got on a luxurious cruise ship called Carnival Valor. It was a magnificent ship with 11 stories. Every facility you could imagine was on board. On the ninth floor there were many restaurants with a wide variety of cuisines from different countries. There were so many choices and many different offerings, from breakfast to lunch to dinner.

The group I traveled with and I were on the second dinner seating. There were many forms of entertainment with different shows each evening; live music, comedies, interactive activities, films and even plays. I did not feel like I was on board a ship; it felt more like a city!

There were over 3,000 people on board the ship. I was traveling with a group of 450 marketers who run their own internet businesses. During one of our activities, we each had two minutes to present our line of business, the method of advertising we utilized, and our results. We had fun exchanging ideas and getting to know one another.

This group did a lot of activities together when we went ashore. We visited Mexico and stopped at the Caribbean islands, The Bahamas, and St. Antonio. I met a lot of new people and made friends that took my mind away from my cancer. I enjoyed every minute!

One day I met another woman who had the same cancer I did. She had just finished her treatment and her husband brought her on the cruise to take her mind off her ordeal and to be among people. We had an obvious, immediate bond and enjoyed sharing our stories in a positive way with each other. It was so nice to talk with someone who knew exactly what I had experienced. We were literally and figuratively in the same boat!

After the cruise, I flew to Tampa, Florida to visit with a friend before flying back to the UK. I was so inspired after the cruise that, once home, I researched alternative treatments and subscribed to cancer research institutes and health science institutes. This led me to various studies and further research on natural treatments for cancer that boast an 80-95% success rate.

MY LIFESTYLE CHANGES

I changed my diet completely and chose to follow Dr. Budwig's diet. I cut down on eating chicken, turkey, and dairy products (except for cottage cheese). I had not eaten red meat since 1986, but in the Budwig Diet you can have red meat every now and then, provided the animal is grass-fed. I continued to carry on eating freshly ground flax seeds, either with vegetable soup or mixed with quark or cottage cheese.

I also began making my own vegetable juices, using mainly organic spinach, kale, carrots, and lettuce. I ate a lot of salads and fresh fruits, including many berries: blueberries, raspberries, strawberries, and black currants. I also eat a lot of red grapes, apples, apricots, and red plums.

I bought lots of books and articles on published research about natural treatments that use diet. I have since met many people who are alive and have been cancer free for 20 years who eschewed chemo and radiation in favor of using their diet as treatment. This is, of course, a personal choice for each individual to make as each person's experiences, treatments, and outcomes will be different.

In addition to the changes I mentioned, I also eliminated sugar and artificial sweeteners; instead, I use natural stevia. I avoid many starches and carbohydrates, eating only small amounts of whole grain breads and pastas. I suggest that you avoid ready-made meals as they are usually full of preservatives. I also recommend that you avoid genetically modified foods and conventionally processed meats as the animals are often given antibiotics and fed dried foods with chemicals. I fear that these additives could cause cancer. Instead, I choose to serve fresh vegetables and organic chicken, fish, or beef.

I have since made long-term changes to my diet because I believe it may prevent my cancer from occurring again. I recently became a vegetarian and I am loving it!

In addition to diet changes, I employed other lifestyle changes as well. I try to avoid stress and worrying. That is much easier said than done! I remember how stressful it was when I discovered the mark on my breast and then later when I heard that I had cancer. Most people will remember how they felt when they were told they have cancer.

Each one of us experiences similar feelings, but each one has his or her own method for dealing with the stress and anxiety, particularly those with young children. You may experience many different emotions during your cancer diagnosis, treatment, and recovery. You may be frightened about what the future will bring to you and the effect it will have on your family. You may feel shocked and angry, as I did, but relieved to know that there is treatment available. If cancer is found and treated early, it may not be the end of your life.

There is much enjoyment to be had in life after cancer treatment. Be positive and think of a bright future ahead of you. Enjoying life to the fullest will help your progress. Have faith and believe that you will conquer cancer and live a normal life!

STRESS, DEPRESSION, AND ANXIETY

It is natural to have feelings of anxiety and/or depression when you are coping with a potentially life-threatening illness. It would be strange if you did not have these feelings! It is how you deal with it that is so important; each one of us has a way to cope with the stress and anxiety.

Anxiety can have many physical and emotional effects, from irritability, moodiness, mood swings, difficulty making decisions, memory loss, fatigue, depression, loss of appetite, and insomnia. Physical signs can include muscle tension, tightness in the chest, a racing heartbeat, and hyperventilation. When these symptoms occur simultaneously, it is called a panic attack.

I experienced most of these during my cancer treatment, but I did my best to prevent anxiety from having a drastic effect on me. I believe the cause of my cancer was the stress I had over the years before the cancer appeared. Today, I do my best to avoid any stress, which is sometimes difficult.

Stress may play a role in the onset of many diseases, particularly cancer, heart problems, and mental illnesses. Stress may reduce your life expectancy and may damage your relationship with your partner and people around you. Anxiety and stress are emotionally devastating and can lead to long-term mental illness. A study published by the American Medical Association in 2008 revealed that anxiety and stress, left untreated, can impair key areas in the brain and cause the symptoms I mentioned above. When we are stressed there will be a shortage of serotonin and Gaba compound in the body. These compounds are the body's natural anxiety and stress relievers, acting as a speed limit for the frenzied communication in the brain. Ignoring stress by brushing it under the rug and hoping it will go away on its own will not work.

When you find that anxious thoughts are taking over and preventing you from focusing on your daily life or affecting your relationship with your loved ones and the people around you, then you need to seek the help of professional people. Do not blame yourself, it is not your fault; many people feel this way. If this happens, you need to seek help from professional people. Ask your doctor to refer you to a counseling service. Most of the time it is easier to talk to a counselor rather than your family and friends. You can tell the counselor exactly how you feel without a filter and they will listen and show you empathy. They will be able to ask questions, perhaps to recall a happy memory or event, to distract you from your negative thoughts and put a smile on your face. Over time this can change the state of your mind by interrupting the negative patterns. to.

Your doctor may suggest antidepressants. I do not accept antidepressants for long-term usage. I believe that they are okay for short term usage, as you are going through a particularly stressful event, but they can be addictive and sometimes cause suicidal thoughts. There is no medical cure for anxiety or depression, only treatments. I believe you need to seek help from a qualified counselor, consider altering your diet, and make changes to your lifestyle.

TIPS FOR COPING WITH STRESS

If you continue to worry about the cancer coming back, your body may produce the same kind of stress hormone as if this were really happening. These stress hormones can cause your mind to be more anxious which results in a vicious cycle that can be difficult to break. There are several things you can do for yourself to cope with stress in addition to seeking professional help. Many of the following suggestions are simple things you can easily do for yourself, yet many of us never think of doing them. I hope you will refer to this list anytime you are feeling anxious, stress, or depressed.

- **Find a hobby:** First of all, it is important to have a healthy distraction, such as a hobby. If you do not currently have a hobby you enjoy, find one! Think of things that interest you that you can incorporate into your life, such as painting. For me, while I am painting, I shut out all negative thoughts and feelings as I focus only on what I am doing.

- **Breathing:** When you feel anxious and stressed, sit down, and take deep breaths. Inhale and exhale slowly 20 times. Imagine each intake of oxygen carrying peace and serenity to all areas of your body. With each exhale, imagine all anxiety and stress leaving your body. Accept that you cannot control everything around you. Do not aim for perfection all the time.

- **Laugh:** It has been said that laughter is the best medicine. So, watch a comedy program on television or buy tickets to see a comic perform. Welcome humor into your life; a good laugh takes your mind away from your worries.

- **Avoid negativity:** Conversely, do not invite other people's stress into your life. Do not watch the news, especially late at night. If you have a friend or family member who brings stress to you, speak with them about it. Remind them that you are in treatment or recovery and do not need any added stress. Accept that you cannot solve the world's problem. Maintain a positive attitude as you replace negative thoughts with positive thoughts.

- **Volunteer:** A terrific way to fill your mind with positive thoughts is to volunteer in your community. Helping others makes you a valuable member of the community and gives you a purpose in life. Focusing on others takes the focus off yourself and your trials. You will feel so rewarded each time you do this!

- **Find a confidante:** Talk to a friend, family member, or even someone at work. You may find a sympathetic, listening ear among your colleagues. It may be helpful for a supportive colleague to be aware of what you are going through. Talk to a member of your family or a close friend when you need to vent about your feelings or your worries. Do not get upset if friends and family tell you to just be positive and pull yourself together. Keep in mind they are simply trying to help and are probably feeling quite helpless. They will not know how you really feel; no one knows except yourself.

- **Tea time:** Drink an herbal team, such as chamomile. In addition to the calming effects of chamomile tea, the ceremony of making and drinking tea will bring about relaxation. Once it becomes a habit, you may find yourself looking forward to your cup of tea and the relaxation it brings. Drinking herbal tea before bed may promote restful sleep.

- **Visualization and meditation:** Visualization and meditation, used separately or together, will reduce stress and tension, relax the mind and body, and improve wellbeing. Lie down or sit comfortably with both feet on the floor, inhale slowly to the count of five and exhale to the count of five. Focus your attention on breathing deeply into your belly. Feel where the breath is going in your body and notice the sensation of breathing out again. For example visualize yourself lying on the beach. Now add your five senses to the picture you have created in your mind. You see the beauty of the sun, sand, and surf. Spend some time here as you picture each detail of the beach. What are you wearing? How many clouds are in the sky? Are there palm trees nearby? Once you have a vivid image of what you see, move on to what you hear. Notice the sounds of the waves crashing on the shore and the seagulls calling to each other. You are breathing the fresh air and smelling the coconut sunscreen you put on your body. You taste the saltiness of the air on your lips. Feel the gentle warmth of the sun shining on your body and the coolness of the sand underneath you. Throughout the visualization, continue your slow, steady breath. Remember to focus on breathing deeply and attend to where the breath is going in your body. If you are feeling too overwhelmed to do a full visualization on your own, listen to a relaxation podcast, calming music, or a recording of natural sounds, such as rainfall, birds singing, or ocean waves.

- **Go for a walk:** Choose a visually appealing location you enjoy and go for a brisk walk. Make it a part of your everyday routine to walk for 30 minutes or more. It will keep you fit, helping your circulation and keeping your heart healthy. You will come to look forward to your daily walk!

- **Practice yoga or Tai-Chi:** Both Tai-Chi and yoga will improve your muscle tone, flexibility, circulation, etc., while promoting relaxation and a feeling of wellbeing.

- **Eat a healthy diet:** I know I have mentioned diet previously, but I cannot emphasize enough how important it is. Unhealthy foods, smoking, and alcohol can all exacerbate stress. Many people think these things calm their stress, but it is just the opposite! Additionally, an unhealthy diet may cause other health issues. Not all alcohol is bad. A glass of red wine occasionally with the evening meal helps you relax and makes you feel sleepy. Red wine is rich in antioxidants which are beneficial to your wellbeing. Do some research to find a red wine rich with resveratrol, a beneficial antioxidant.

- **Complementary therapies:** In addition to the coping strategies for dealing with stress, there are several other complementary therapies. These may be used alongside other treatments and include aromatherapy, reflexology, massage, music therapy, reiki, and acupuncture, to name a few.

A FAVORITE RECIPE

I have decided to share one of my personal recipes with you. This is the salad I have every day, with lunch and dinner, throughout summer and winter. I never get bored with it. I alternate some of the ingredients and buy varieties of lettuce according to the season and availability.

Yvonne's Herbal Salad

Ingredients:

- 4 leaves of lettuce (I recommend Romaine or whatever lettuce is in season where you live)

- 4 small radishes

- ¼ of a cucumber

- ½ small red onion or other onion

- 100 gm of rocket (also called arugula)

- 1 small boiled beetroot

- A few leaves of fresh mint or dried mint

- ½ freshly squeezed lemon

- 1 clove of garlic minced or chopped

- 3 tablespoon of extra virgin olive oil or organic flaxseed oil

- A pinch of salt

Method:

1. Wash all lettuces and vegetables under cool running water.

2. Chop the lettuce, radish, cucumber, rocket, beetroot, and onion and place in a bowl.

3. Mix the mint, lemon, garlic, oil, and salt together. Pour over the vegetables and enjoy.

Additions and Alterations:

Occasionally, maybe once a month, I add 40 gm of feta cheese to the salad. Other times I may add black olives. I sometimes change up the vegetables I use, depending on what is in season. I may use baby-leaf spinach mixed with rocket and omit the cucumber. I sometimes add a small tomato and grated carrot. I may use fresh thyme or dill, when in season.

I also like to add freshly boiled red kidney beans on occasion. I soak dried beans overnight and boil in the morning to use in my salad later in the day. (I never buy tin food, as it is full of sugar, salt, and preservatives.)

Other times I use boiled chickpeas in the salad. Or, I make them as a dip to enjoy on the side. I mash the chickpeas with added lemon juice, olive or flaxseed oil, garlic, onion, and mint. I enjoy this as a side with my salad.

I concluded that what you eat matters to your health to maintain your immune system and lead a healthy life. I hope you enjoy this recipe and that it inspires you to create other healthy options. If you would like to have more recipes and learn what to eat and do to remain healthy, build your immune system, and boost your energy, send me an email at naderyvonne@ yahoo.com

Branding Small Business

RAYMOND AARON

B randing is an incredibly important tool for creating and building your business. Large companies have been benefiting from branding ever since people first started selling things to other people. Branding made those businesses big.

If you're a small business owner, you probably imagine that small companies are different and don't need branding as much as large companies do. Not true. The truth is small businesses need branding just as much, if not more, than large companies.

Perhaps you've thought about branding, but assumed you'd need millions of dollars to do it properly, or that branding is just the same thing as marketing. Nothing could be further from the truth.

Marketing is the engine of your company's success. Branding is the fuel in that engine.

In the old days, salespeople were a big part of the selling process. They recommended one product over another and laid out the reasons why it was better. Salespeople had credibility because they knew about all the products, and customers often took the advice they had to offer.

Today, consumers control the buying process. They shop in big box stores, super-sized supermarkets, and over the Internet — where there are no salespeople. Buyers now get online and gather information beforehand. They learn about all the products available and look to see if there really is any difference between them. Consumers also read reviews and check social media to see if both the company and the product are reputable. In other words, they want to know what the brand is all about.

The way of commerce used to be: "Nothing happens till something is sold." Today it's: "Nothing happens till something is branded!"

DEFINING A BRAND

A brand is a proper name that stands for something. It lives in the consumer's mind, has positive or negative characteristics, and invokes a feeling or an image. In short, it's a person's perception of a product or a company.

When all goes well, consumers associate the same characteristics with a brand that the company talks about in its advertising, public relations, marketing and sales materials. Of course, when a product doesn't live up to what the company says about it, the brand gets a bad reputation. On the other hand, if a product or service over-delivers on the promises made, the brand can become a superstar.

RECOGNIZING BRANDING AND ITS CHARACTERISTICS

Branding is the science and art of making something that isn't unique, unique. Branding in the marketplace is the same as branding on a ranch. On a ranch, ranchers use branding to differentiate their cattle from every other rancher's cattle (because all cattle look pretty much the same). In the marketplace, branding is what makes a product stand out in a crowd of similar products. The right branding gets you noticed, remembered and sold — or perhaps I should say bought, because today it is all about buying, not selling.

There are four main characteristics of branding that make it an integral part of the marketing and purchasing process.

1. Branding makes you trustworthy and known

Branding makes a product more special than other products. With branding, a normal, everyday product has a personality, and a first and last name, and people know who you are.

In today's marketplace, most products are, more or less, just like their competition. Toilet paper is toilet paper, milk is milk, and a grocery store by any other name is still a grocery store. However, branding takes a product and makes it unique. For example, high-quality drinking water is available from just about every tap in the Western world and it's free, but people pay good money for it when it comes in a bottle. Branding takes bottled water and makes Evian.

Furthermore, every aspect of your brand gives potential customers a feeling or comfort level that they associate with you. The more powerful and positive that feeling is, the more easily and more frequently they will want to do business with you and, indeed, will do business with you.

2. Branding differentiates you from others

Strong branding makes you better than your competition, and makes your product name memorable and easy to remember. Even if your product is absolutely the same as every other product like it, branding makes it special. Branding makes it the first product a consumer thinks about when deciding to make a purchase.

Branding also makes a product seem popular. Everyone knows about it, which implicitly says people like it. And, if people like it, it must be good.

3. Branding makes you worth more money

The stronger your branding is, the more likely people are willing to spend that little bit extra because they believe you, your product, your service, or your business are worth it. They may say they won't, but they will. They do it all the time.

For example, a one-pound box of Godiva chocolates costs about $40; the same weight of Hershey's Kisses costs about $4. The quality of the chocolate isn't ten times greater. The reason people buy Godiva is that the brand Godiva means "gift" whereas the brand Hershey means "snack". Gifts obviously cost more than snacks.

4. Branding pre-sells your product

In the buying age, people most often make the decision on which products to pick up before they walk into the store. The stronger the branding, the more likely people are to think in terms of your product rather than the product category. For example, people are as likely, maybe even more likely, to add Hellmann's to the shopping list as they are to write down simply mayo. The same is true for soda, ketchup, and many other products with successful, strong branding.

Plus, as soon as a shopper gets to the shelf, branding can provide a quick reminder of what products to grab in a few ways:

- An icon or logo
- A specific color
- An audio icon

BRANDING IN A SMALL BUSINESS

Big companies spend millions of dollars on advertising, marketing, and public relations (PR) to build recognition of a new product name. They get their selling messages out to the public using television, radio, magazines, and the Internet. They can even throw money at damage control when necessary. The strategies for branding are the same in a small business, but the scale, costs, and a few of the tactics change.

Make your brand name work harder

The name of a small business can mean everything in terms of branding. Your brand name needs to work harder for your business than you do. It's the first thing a prospective customer sees, and it is how they will remember you. A brand name has to be memorable when spoken, and focused in its meaning. If the name doesn't represent what consumers believe about a product and the company that makes it, then that brand will fail.

In building your product's reputation and image, less is often significantly more. Make sure the name you choose immediately gives a sense of what you do.

Large corporations have millions of dollars to take a meaningless brand name and make it stand for something. Small businesses don't, so use words that really mean something. Strive for something interesting and be right on point. You don't need to be boring.

Plumbers, for example, would do well setting themselves apart with names like "The On-Time Plumber" or "24/7 Plumbing". The same is true for electricians, IT providers, or even marketing consultants. Plenty of other types of business are so general in nature they just don't work hard enough in a business or product name.

Even the playing field: The Net

The Internet has leveled the playing field for small businesses like nothing else. You can use the Internet in several ways to market your brand:

Website: Developing and maintaining a website is easier than ever. Anyone can find your business regardless of its size.

Social Media: Facebook and Twitter can promote your brand in a cost-effective manner.

BUILDING YOUR BRAND WITH THE BRANDING LADDER

Even if you do everything perfectly the first time (and I don't know anyone who does), branding takes time. How much time isn't just up to you, but you can speed things along by understanding the different levels of branding, as well as the business and marketing strategies that can get you to the top.

Introducing the Branding Ladder

Moving through the levels of branding is like climbing a ladder to the top of the marketplace. The Branding Ladder has five distinct rungs and, unlike stairs, you can't take them two at a time. You have to take them in order, and some businesses spend more time on each rung than others.

You can also think of the Branding Ladder in terms of a scale from zero to ten. Everyone starts at zero. If you properly climb the ladder, you can end up at 12 out of 10. The Branding Ladder below shows a special rung at the top of the ladder that can take your business over the top. The following section explains the Branding Ladder and how your small business can move up it.

THE BRANDING LADDER	
Brand Advocacy	12/10
Brand Insistence	10/10
Brand Preference	3/10
Brand Awareness	1/10
Brand Absence	0/10

Rung 1: Living in the void

Your business, in fact every business, starts at the bottom rung, which is called brand absence, meaning you have no brand whatsoever except your own name. On a scale of one to ten, brand absence is, of course, zero. That's the worst place to live and obviously the most difficult entrepreneurially. The good news is that the only way is up.

Ninety-seven percent of businesses live on this rung of the Branding Ladder. They earn far less than they want to earn, far less than they should earn, and far less than they would earn if they did exactly the same work under a real brand.

Rung 2: Achieving awareness

Brand awareness is a good first step up the ladder to the second rung. Actually, it's really good, especially because 97 percent of businesses never get there. You want people to be aware of you. When person A speaks to person B and says, "Have you heard of "The 24/7 Plumber?" You want the answer to be "yes".

On that scale of one to ten, however, brand awareness is only a one. It's better than nothing, but not that much better. Although people know of your brand, being aware doesn't mean that they are interested in buying it. Coca Cola drinkers know about Pepsi, but they don't drink it.

Rung 3: Becoming the preferred brand

Getting to the third rung, brand preference, is definitely a real step up. This rung means that people prefer to use your product or service rather than that of your competition. They believe there is a real difference between you and others, and you're their first choice. This rung is a crucial branding stage for parity products, such as bottled water and breakfast cereals, not to mention plumbers, electricians, lawyers, and all the others. Brand preference is clearly better than brand awareness, but it's less than halfway up the ladder.

Car rental companies represent a perfect example of why brand preference may not be enough. When someone lands at an airport and needs to rent a car on the spot, he or she may go straight to the preferred rental counter. If that company has a car available, it's a sale. However, if all the cars for that company have been rented, the person will move to the next rental kiosk without much thought, because one rental car is just as good as another.

Exerting Brand Preference needs to be easy and convenient

If all you have is brand preference, your business is on shaky ground and you can lose business for the feeblest of reasons. Very few people go to a second or third supermarket just to find their favorite brand of bottled water. Similarly, a shopper may prefer one store over another but, if both stores sell the same products, he or she will often go to the closest store even if it is not the better liked one. The reason for staying nearby does not need to be a dramatic one — the shopper may simply be tired, on a tight schedule, or not in the mood to travel.

Rung 4: Making it you and only you

When your customers are so committed to your product or service that they won't accept a substitute, you have reached the fourth rung of the Branding Ladder. All companies strive to reach this place, called brand insistence.

Brand insistence means that someone's experience with a product in terms of performance, durability, customer service, and image has been sufficiently exceptional. As a result, the product has earned an incredible level of loyalty.

If the product isn't available where the customer is, he or she will literally not buy something else. Rather, the person will look for the preferred product elsewhere. Can you imagine what a fabulous place this is for a company to be? Brand insistence is the best of the best, the perfect ten out of ten, the whole ball of wax.

Apple is a perfect example of brand insistence

Apple users don't just think, they know in their heads and hearts, that anything made by Apple is technologically-advanced, user-friendly, and just all-around superior. Committed to everything Apple, Mac users won't even entertain the thought that a PC may have positive attributes.

Apple people love everything about their Macs, iPads, iPhones, the Mac stores and all those apps. When the company introduces a new product, many of its brand-insistent fans actually wait in line overnight to be one of the first to have it. Steve Jobs is one of their idols.

Considering one big potential problem

Unfortunately, you can lose brand insistence much more quickly than you can achieve it. Brand-insistent customers have such high expectations that they can be disillusioned or disappointed by just one bad product experience. You also have to consistently reinforce the positives because insistence can fade over time. Even someone who has bought and re-bought a specific brand of car for the last 20 years can decide it's just time for a change. That's how fickle the world is.

At ten out of ten, brand insistence may seem like the top rung of the ladder, but it's not. One rung is actually better, and it involves getting your brand-insistent customers to keep polishing your brand for you.

Rung 5: Getting customers to do the work for you

Brand advocacy is the highest rung on the ladder. It's better than ten out of ten because you have customers who are so happy with your product that they want everyone to know about it and use it. Think of them as uber-fans. Not only do they recommend you to friends and family, they also practically shout your praises from the rooftops, interrupt conversations among strangers to give their opinion, and tell everyone they meet how fantastic you are. Most companies can only aspire to this level of customer satisfaction. Apple is one of the few large corporations in recent history that has brand advocates all over the world.

- Brand advocacy does the following five extraordinary things for your company. Brand advocacy:

- Provides a level of visibility that you couldn't pay for if you tried. Brand advocates are so enthusiastic they talk about you all the time, and reach people in ways general media and public relations can't. You get great visibility because they make sure people actually listen.

- Delivers free advertising and public relations. Companies love the extra super-positive messaging, all for free.

- Affords a level of credibility that literally can't be bought. Brand advocates are more than just walking testimonials. They are living proof that you are the best.

- Provides pre-sold prospective customers. Advocate recommendations carry so much weight that they are worth much more than plain referrals. They deliver customers ready and committed to purchasing your product or service.

- Increases profits exponentially. Brand advocates are money-making machines for your business because they increase sales and decrease marketing costs.

For these reasons, brand advocacy is 12 out of 10!!

BRANDING YOURSELF: HOW TO DO SO IN FOUR EASY WAYS

If you're interested in branding your product or company, you may not be sure where to begin. The good news: I'm here to help. You can brand in many ways, but here I pare it down to four ways to help you start:

Branding by association

This way involves hanging out with and being seen with people who are very much higher than you in your particular niche.

Branding by achievement

This way repurposes your previous achievements.

Branding by testimonial

This way makes use of the testimonials that you receive but have likely never used.

Branding by WOW

A WOW is the pleasantly unexpected, the equivalent of going the extra mile. The easiest and most certain way to WOW people is to tell them that you've written a book. To discover how you can write a book of own, go to www.BrandingSmallBusinessForDummies.com.

Happiness: How to Experience the "Real Deals"

MARCI SHIMOFF

I was 41 years old, stretched out on a lounge chair by my pool and reflecting on my life. I had achieved all that I thought I needed to be happy.

You see, when I was a child, I thought there would be five main things that would ensure that I'd be happy: a successful career helping people, a loving husband, a comfortable home, a great body, and a wonderful circle of friends. After years of study, hard work, and a few "lucky breaks," I finally had them all. (Okay, so my body didn't quite look like Halle Berry's—but four out of five isn't bad!) You think I'd have been on the top of the world.

But surprisingly I wasn't. I felt an emptiness inside that the outer successes of life couldn't fill. I was also afraid that if I lost any of those things, I might be miserable. Sadly, I knew I wasn't alone in feeling this way.

While happiness is the one thing we all truly want, so few people really experience the deep and lasting fulfillment that fills our soul. Why aren't we finding it?

Because, in the words of the old country western song, we're looking for happiness in "all the wrong places."

Looking around, I saw that the happiest people I knew weren't the most successful and famous. Some were married, some were single. Some had lots of money, and some didn't have a dime. Some of them even had health challenges. From where I stood, there seemed to be no rhyme or reason to what made people happy. The obvious question became: *Could a person actually be happy for no reason?*

I had to find out.

So I threw myself into the study of happiness. I interviewed scores of scientists, as well as 100 unconditionally happy people. (I call them the Happy 100.) I delved into the research from the burgeoning field of positive psychology, the study of the positive traits that enable people to enjoy meaningful, fulfilling, and happy lives.

What I found changed my life. To share this knowledge with others, I wrote a book called *Happy for No Reason: 7 Steps to Being Happy from the Inside Out.*

One day, as I sat down to compile my findings, all the pieces of the puzzle fell into place. I had a simple, but profound "a-ha"—there's a continuum of happiness:

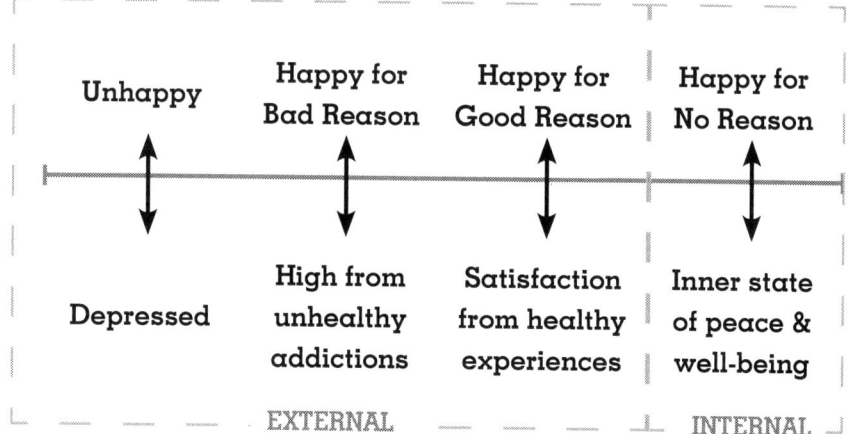

Unhappy: We all know what this means: life seems flat. Some of the signs are anxiety, fatigue, feeling blue or low—your "garden-variety" unhappiness. This isn't the same as clinical depression, which is characterized by deep despair and hopelessness that dramatically interferes with your ability to live a normal life, and for which professional help is absolutely necessary.

Happy for Bad Reason: When people are unhappy, they often try to make themselves feel better by indulging in addictions or behaviors that may feel good in the moment but are ultimately detrimental. They seek the highs that come from drugs, alcohol, excessive sex, "retail therapy," compulsive gambling, over-eating, and too much television-watching, to name a few. This kind of "happiness" is hardly happiness at all. It is only a temporary way to numb or escape our unhappiness through fleeting experiences of pleasure.

Happy for Good Reason: This is what people usually mean by happiness: having good relationships with our family and friends, success in our careers, financial security, a nice house or car, or using our talents and strengths well. It's the pleasure we derive from having the healthy things in our lives that we want.

Don't get me wrong. I'm all for this kind of happiness! It's just that it's only half the story. Being Happy for Good Reason depends on the external conditions of our lives—these conditions change or are lost, our happiness usually goes too. Relying solely on this type of happiness is where a lot of our fear is stemming from these days. We're afraid the things we think we need to be happy may be slipping from our grasp.

Deep inside, I think we all know that life isn't meant to be about getting by, numbing our pain, or having everything "under control." True happiness doesn't come from merely collecting an assortment of happy experiences. At our core, we know there's something more than this.

There is. It's the next level on the happiness continuum—Happy for No Reason.

Happy for No Reason: This is true happiness—a state of peace and well-being that isn't dependent on external circumstances.

Happy for No Reason isn't elation, euphoria, mood spikes, or peak experiences that don't last. It doesn't mean grinning like a fool 24/7 or experiencing a superficial high. Happy for No Reason isn't an emotion. In fact, when you are Happy for No Reason, you can have *any* emotion—including sadness, fear, anger or hurt—but you still experience that underlying state of peace and well-being.

When you're Happy for No Reason, you *bring* happiness to your outer experiences rather than trying to *extract* happiness from them. You don't need to manipulate the world around you to try to make yourself happy. You live from happiness, rather than *for* happiness.

This is a revolutionary concept. Most of us focus on being Happy for Good Reason, stringing together as many happy experiences as we can, like beads in a necklace, to create a happy life. We have to spend a lot of time and energy trying to find just the right beads so we can have a "happy necklace".

Being Happy for No Reason, in our necklace analogy, is like having a happy string. No matter what beads we put on our necklace—good, bad or indifferent—our inner experience, which is the string that runs through them all, is happy, and creates a happy life.

Happy for No Reason is a state that's been spoken of in virtually all spiritual and religious traditions throughout history. The concept is universal. In Buddhism, it is called causeless joy; in Christianity, the kingdom of Heaven within; and in Judaism it is called *ashrei*, an inner sense of holiness and health. In Islam it is called *falah*, happiness and well-being; and in Hinduism it is called *ananda*, or pure bliss. Some traditions refer to it as an enlightened or awakened state.

So how can you be Happy for No Reason?

Science is verifying the way. Researchers in the field of positive psychology have found that we each have a "happiness set-point," that determines our level of happiness. No matter what happens, whether it's something as exhilarating as winning the lottery or as challenging as a horrible accident, most people eventually return to their original happiness level. Like your weight set-point, which keeps the scale hovering around the same number, your happiness set-point will remain the same **unless you make a concerted effort to change it.** In the same way you'd crank up the thermostat to get comfortable on a chilly day, you actually have the power to reprogram your happiness set-point to a higher level of peace and well-being. The secret lies in practicing the habits of happiness.

Some books and programs will tell you that you can simply decide to be happy. They say just make up your mind to be happy—and you will be.

I don't agree.

You can't just decide to be happy, any more than you can decide to be fit or to be a great piano virtuoso and expect instant mastery. You can, however, decide to take the necessary steps, like exercising or taking piano lessons—and by practicing those skills, you can get in shape or give recitals. In the same way, you can become Happy for No Reason through practicing the habits of happy people.

All of your habitual thoughts and behaviors in the past have created specific neural pathways in the wiring in your brain, like grooves in a record. When we think or behave a certain way over and over, the neural pathway is strengthened and the groove becomes deeper—the way a well-traveled route through a field eventually becomes a clear-cut path. Unhappy people tend to have more negative neural pathways. This is why you can't just ignore the realities of your brain's wiring and *decide* to be happy! To raise your level of happiness, you have to create new grooves.

Scientists used to think that once a person reached adulthood, the brain was fairly well "set in stone" and there wasn't much you could do to change it. But new research is revealing exciting information about the brain's neuroplasticity: when you think, feel and act in different ways, the brain changes and actually rewires itself. You aren't doomed to the same negative neural pathways for your whole life. Leading brain researcher Dr. Richard Davidson, of the University of Wisconsin says, "Based on what we know of the plasticity of the brain, we can think of things like happiness and compassion as skills that are no different from learning to play a musical instrument or tennis …. it is possible to train our brains to be happy."

While a few of the Happy 100 I interviewed were born happy, most of them learned to be happy by practicing habits that supported their happiness. That means wherever you are on the happiness continuum, it's entirely in your power to raise your happiness level.

In the course of my research, I uncovered 21 core happiness habits that anyone can use to become happier and stay that way. You can find all 21 happiness habits at www.HappyForNoReason.com

Here are a few tips to get you started:

1. **Incline Your Mind Toward Joy.** Have you noticed that your mind tends to register the negative events in your life more than the positive? If you get ten compliments in a day and one criticism, what do you remember? For most people, it's the criticism. Scientists call this our "negativity bias" — our primitive survival wiring that causes us to pay more attention to the negative than the positive. To reverse this bias, get into the daily habit of consciously registering the positive around you: the sun on your skin, the taste of a favorite food, a smile or kind word from a co-worker or friend. Once you notice something positive, take a moment to savor it deeply and feel it; make it more than just a mental observation. Spend 20 seconds soaking up the happiness you feel.

2. **Let Love Lead.** One way to power up your heart's flow is by sending loving kindness to your friends and family, as well as strangers you pass on the street. Next time you're waiting for the elevator at work, stuck in a line at the store or caught up in traffic, send a silent wish to the people you see for their happiness, well-being, and health. Simply wishing others well switches on the "pump" in your own heart that generates love and creates a strong current of happiness.

3. **Lighten Your Load.** To make a habit of letting go of worries and negative thoughts, start by letting go on the physical level. Cultural anthropologist Angeles Arrien recommends giving or throwing away 27 items a day for nine days. This deceptively simple practice will help you break attachments that no longer serve you.

4. **Make Your Cells Happy.** Your brain contains a veritable pharmacopeia of natural happiness-enhancing neurochemicals — endorphins, serotonin, oxytocin, and dopamine — just waiting to be released to every organ and cell in your body. The way that you eat, move, rest, and even your facial expression can shift the balance of your body's feel-good-chemicals, or "Joy Juice", in your favor. To dispense some extra Joy Juice — smile. Scientists have discovered that smiling decreases stress hormones and boosts happiness chemicals, which increase the body's T-cells, reduce pain, and enhance relaxation. You may not feel like it, but smiling — even artificially to begin with — starts the ball rolling and will turn into a real smile in short order.

5. **Hang with the Happy.** We catch the emotions of those around us just like we catch their colds — it's called emotional contagion. So it's important to make wise choices about the company you keep. Create appropriate boundaries with emotional bullies and "happiness vampires" who suck the life out of you. Develop your happiness "dream team" — a mastermind or support group you meet with regularly to keep you steady on the path of raising your happiness.

"Happily ever after" isn't just for fairytales or for only the lucky few. Imagine experiencing inner peace and well-being as the backdrop for everything else in your life. When you're Happy for No Reason, it's not that your life always looks perfect — it's that, however it looks, you'll still be happy!

By Marci Shimoff. Based on the New York Times bestseller *Happy for No Reason: 7 Steps to Being Happy from the Inside Out*, which offers a revolutionary approach to experiencing deep and lasting happiness. The woman's face of the *Chicken Soup for the Soul* series and a featured teacher in *The Secret*, Marci is an authority on success, happiness, and the law of attraction. To order *Happy for No Reason* and receive free bonus gifts, go to www.happyfornoreason.com/mybook.

Sex, Love and Relationships

DR. JOHN GRAY

Just as great sex is important to lasting love, good health is important to sex and relationships. About 12 years ago, I cured myself of early stage Parkinson's disease. The doctors were amazed, but my wife was even more amazed. She noted that our relationship and sex life had become dramatically better. It turns out that the natural supplements I used to reverse Parkinson's can also make you more attentive and loving in your relationship. At that point, I realized that good relationship skills alone were not enough to sustain love and passion for a lifetime.

I shared many insights gained from my 40 years' experience as a marriage counselor and coach in *Men Are From Mars, Women Are From Venus*. And while my insights go a long way towards helping men and women understand and support each other, good communication skills alone are not always enough. For better relationships, we not only need to be healthy, but we must also experience optimum brain function.

If you are tired, depressed, anxious, not sleeping well, or in pain, then certainly romantic feelings will become a thing of the past. My recovery from Parkinson's revealed to me the profound connection between the quality of our health and our relationships. This insight has motivated me, over the past twelve years, to research the secrets of optimum health as a foundation for lasting love.

These are health secrets that are generally not explored in medical school. In medical school, doctors are indoctrinated into the culture of examining the symptoms, identifying the sickness, and prescribing a drug to treat that sickness. They learn very little about how to be healthy or to sustain successful relationships.

There are no university courses entitled "Better Nutrition For Better Sex". Drugs sometimes save lives, but they also have negative side effects that do little to preserve the passion in a relationship. Ideally, drugs should be used as a last resort and 90 % of our health plan should be drug free. From this perspective, the heath care crisis, as well as our high rate of divorce in America, is indirectly caused by our dependence on doctors and prescription drugs.

Most people have not even considered that taking prescribed drugs (even for the small stuff) can weaken their relationships, which in turn makes them more vulnerable to more disease. For example, if you are feeling depressed or anxious, a drug may numb your pain, but it does nothing to help you correct the cause of your problem. It can even prevent you from feeling your natural motivation to get the emotional support you need. In a variety of ways, our common health complaints are all expressions of two major conditions: our lack of education to identify and support unmet gender-specific emotional needs; and our lack of education to identify and support unmet gender-specific nutritional needs.

With an understanding of natural solutions that have been around for thousands of years, drugs are not needed to treat many common complaints. Some symptoms like low energy, weight gain, allergies, hormonal imbalance, mood swings, poor sleep, indigestion, lack of focus, ADD and ADHD, procrastination, low motivation, memory loss, decreased libido, PMS, vaginal dryness, muscle and joint pain, or the lack of passion in life and/or our relationships can be treated drug-free. By using drugs (even over-the-counter drugs) to treat these common complaints, our bodies and relationships are weakened, making us more vulnerable to bigger and more costly health challenges like cancer, diabetes, heart disease, auto-immune disease, dementia, and Alzheimer's. In simple terms, by handling the easy stuff (the common complaints) without doctors and drugs, we can protect ourselves from the big stuff (cancer, heart disease, dementia, etc.) We can be healthy and also enjoy lasting love and passion in our personal lives.

Even if you are taking anti-depressants or hormone replacement therapy, sometimes all it takes to stop treating the symptom is to directly handle the cause. With specific mineral orotates (something most people have never heard of) or omega three oil from the brains of salmon, your stress levels immediately drop and you begin to feel happy and in love again.

For every health challenge, we have explored the effects on our relationships, with as well as natural remedies that can sometimes produce immediate positive results. You can find these natural solutions to common health complaints for free at my website: www.MarsVenus.com.

What they don't teach in medical school is how to be healthy and happy without the use of drugs or hormone replacement. By refusing drugs and taking responsibility for your health, a wealth of new possibilities can become available to you. We are designed to be healthy and happy, and it is within our reach if we commit to increasing our knowledge.

New research regarding the brain differences in men and women reveals how specific nutritional supplements, combined with gender-specific relationship and self-nurturing skills, can stimulate the hormones of health, happiness and increased energy. Over the past 10 years in my healing center in California, I witnessed how natural solutions coupled with gender-specific relationship skills could solve our common health complaints without drugs. By addressing these common complaints without prescribed drugs, not only do we feel better, but our relationships have the potential to improve dramatically.

Ultimately the cause of all our common complaints is higher stress levels. Researchers around the world all agree that chronic stress levels in our bodies provide a basis for any and all disease to take hold. An easy and quick solution for lowering our stress reactions is specific nutritional support combined with gender-smart relationship skills. Extra nutritional support is needed because stress depletes the body very quickly of essential nutrients. When a car engine is running more quickly, it uses fuel more quickly. When we are stressed, we need both extra nutrients and extra emotional support. Understanding what we need to take and where to get it requires education. Every week day at www.MarsVenus.com I have a live daily show where I freely answer questions and provide this much-needed new gender-specific insight.

At www.MarsVenus.com, we are happy to share what we have learned for creating healthy bodies and positive relationships. You can find a host of natural solutions for common complaints and feel confident that you have the power to feel fully alive with an abundance of energy and positive feelings that will enrich all your relationships.

Simple Steps for Big Results in Boosting Heart Health

RALSTON POWELL

"First say to yourself what you would be: and then do what you have to do."
— Epictetus

I t strikes like lightning, and it steals loved ones from their families. It is the number one killer of men and women in Western societies; twelve million people die from it each year around the world. While some of its warning signs are obvious, it can come disguised as flu, headache, or just plain fatigue.

Some people have no symptoms and do not see it coming. They are oblivious to the damage that is already done until they are at severe risk of a catastrophe. It can happen at any time, even when they are at rest. If you do not act fast enough or seek help within minutes, it can be fatal.

What am I talking about here? What is this disease that takes lives by stealth, which can recur even when you've recovered from it?

A heart attack.

How many of you have lost a loved one, a friend, or a colleague to a heart attack? Sadly enough, there are many of us in these ranks. It is clear that people are getting sick and dying even at a young age. In fact, I first became concerned about the rising incidence of both heart disease and cancer when a member of my church died of Leukemia. This man was young, approximately 30 years old with a wife and young children. At the time, anyone who was diagnosed with cancer of the blood felt a sense of hopelessness. The second time I felt a sense of concern was when I heard of the death of a young man at a prominent company that I would visit daily. His diagnosis was a massive heart attack. Following that, a friend and co-worker who was having problems with his heart went on vacation to Guyana; in the heat, he suffered a massive heart attack and died. These experiences made me concerned enough to do research, and I found out that heart disease is stated to be North America's number one killer. People from all walks of life can be affected.

Heart disease is commonly reported among those who are physically unfit, carry too much weight, who smoke and drink heavily, and who are eating fat-rich foods. Yet it is no longer just the plight of middle-aged men. Women are just as susceptible, especially after menopause.

Tragically, there are now stories that heart disease is striking the seemingly healthy. You can be a marathon runner, observe a low-calorie diet, have manageable cholesterol, and you can still suffer a catastrophic heart attack without any notice or warning signs.

WHAT IS A HEART ATTACK?

Your heart is no bigger than a fist, but it is your strongest organ, and it works tirelessly from the time you take your first breath to your last. It is made of cardiac muscle, a specialized muscle that only exists in the heart, and, unlike muscles in our legs or arms, the cardiac muscle never tires.

The heart works to pump life-giving oxygen and nutrients in the blood to every part of your body. On average, it beats between 60-100 times per minute at rest. When you work out or are feeling anxious or angry, your heart beats more quickly.

Feeding the heart with blood are the coronary arteries. When there is too much cholesterol in the bloodstream, it gets deposited on the inner linings of these blood vessels, just like rust on the insides of old plumbing. These deposits, called plaque, build up and block oxygen from getting to the heart.

Decreased blood flow causes chest pain, angina, or shortness of breath. A complete blockage of blood flow can damage or destroy part of the heart muscle. Typical symptoms of an attack are anxiety, sweating, chest pain, stiffness or discomfort in the upper body, nausea, and stomach pain.

A person can survive a heart attack due, in part, to significant improvements in medical treatment, yet the statistics are ugly. More than 60% of people who suffer a heart attack die before getting the medical help that they need.

WHAT'S THE GOOD NEWS HERE?

The good news is that a heart attack is absolutely preventable. And its damage is reversible. If you've suffered the disease before, you can empower yourself to make sure you'll never be victim to another attack again. You can do so with minimal or zero drug use or surgical interventions, such as a coronary bypass or having stents placed in your arteries to improve blood flow.

You can lead a healthier life by making easy lifestyle changes. These adjustments are so simple you can see results within a month. Not only that, but you also reduce the risks against you by more than half.

Pretty good news, isn't it?

Changing the way you live is far more effective in prevention and repair than any number of drugs or tubes put into your body. Treating only the symptoms or the risks is taking the short-view, and that is why, once your doctor prescribes medication, you are on it for the rest of your life. You can stop playing the victim and take back control of your own life. By investing some time and committing to making the changes, you can protect yourself from this devastating disease and live life fully.

HEALTH IS OUR BIRTHRIGHT

It is time for a paradigm shift in the way we look at the prevention of heart disease and its therapy for rehabilitation. We must go beyond the conventional attitudes and treatments that limit how we can live healthier lives.

The first step we must take is to change the way we look at our health. I've always firmly believed that health is our birthright. Our bodies are wonderful, complex, finely-tuned instruments. There're no two ways of saying it - it is a miracle!

Picture this. You make a small cut on your finger when you're cutting vegetables. You may run tap water over the finger to stop the bleeding, pour hydrogen peroxide on it, and apply a band-aid. Since it was a small and superficial cut, you're completely healed within a few days. Voila!

But what has taken place without conscious intervention from you is a sequence of healing events. The moment the skin is cut, the blood vessels feeding blood to the area miraculously reduce blood flow to the injured area, like turning off the tap. Next, platelets rush to the scene. They have been alerted to the emergency by enzymes released from the damaged blood vessels. The platelets clot together to form a plug that becomes a scab to stop the blood vessel from bleeding further. In the meantime, signals are sent out to more platelets to come help at the site of the damage.

When the bleeding is under control, the constricted blood vessels open up again, this time bringing important white blood cells to destroy any germs or infections that may have gotten into the body through the wound. Then the body concentrates on healing and rebuilding. The skin on both sides of the cut stretches to meet in the middle, forming a scar, which may or may not disappear as the body adds more collagen to the area. The finger is almost as good as new.

Notice that I said all of this happened without any conscious thought on your part. That's because you are gifted with a terrific immune system with enormous healing power, which orchestrates events to repair and renew your body even as you're reading this sentence.

TIME TO GET SMART ABOUT HEART HEALTH

Why does disease happen then? When we are out of balance, both physically and emotionally, we suppress our immune functions. We turn our body from its natural alkaline state in which disease cannot flourish to an acidic state, which is ripe ground for illnesses like heart diseases and diabetes.

We need to look at health as being much more than just being free of disease. We should look at health as the perfect mind-body balance and the platform from which we can reach our highest potential, our greatest creativity, and lasting happiness.

At this point, I wish to reiterate that power lies within you.

What if there is a history of heart disease in your family? Doesn't it run in the genes? It is mistaken thinking to blame it on a shared heritage. Heart attacks are caused by how the environment affects your genes. So, really, it is what you eat, how much or little you exercise, how you handle stress, and environmental toxins that cause hypertension, high cholesterol, and other imbalances such as high blood sugar that increase the risk of a heart attack.

By turning from victim to someone who takes control with courage and determination, you will make healthy choices, add beneficial foods, exercises, therapies, and natural supplements to your lifestyle. Remember to be kind to yourself and take baby steps, but also congratulate yourself for every accomplishment, no matter how small.

CUT BACK RISK FACTORS

The number of things that make us more vulnerable to heart attacks are called risk factors. Research shows that poor lifestyle choices heighten some of these risk factors, including:

- Smoking
- Unhealthy diet

- Insufficient exercise
- Chronic stress

These unfortunate lifestyle decisions lead to physical problems such as high blood pressure, high blood sugar, and a high level of blood fats. High blood pressure forces the heart to work harder than it should, causing it to weaken faster over time. High blood sugar speeds up the narrowing and the hardening of the arteries. We have already discussed the damage to the heart from high cholesterol levels.

Unrelieved stress from feeling anxious, lonely, isolated, or angry also causes significant damage. It is hard to accept that stress can be the single trigger for a heart attack. But stress creates that string of events that can lead to that one, catastrophic heart attack. Stress raises cholesterol levels, aggravates blood sugar imbalances, and elevates blood pressure, all of which make the blood more likely to clot.

In plain speak, the more risk factors there are in your life, the higher the risk you run of a heart attack.

SIMPLE STEPS, BIG RESULTS

There are steps you can take, starting now. It is better for you to add one simple change every day rather than attempt to do everything at once and give up down the road because you're overwhelmed by having to do too much at any one time.

Here are a few suggestions of what you can do:

1. Stop smoking. You reduce the odds of a heart attack from the very moment you stop using tobacco.

2. Move it, move it, move it. Medical literature recommends exercising 30 minutes or more several days of the week. But in a pinch, even ten minutes of intense physical exercise goes a long way to making a difference. Take the stairs rather than the escalator, take a walk during lunch, get off at an earlier stop and walk the last few blocks to work or home.

3. Eat heart-healthy foods. Five servings of fruit and vegetables are a daily must, and if you must snack, pick vegetables like carrots, cucumbers, peppers, or fruit. Avoid the temptation to indulge in a sugar-rich pastry. Other heart-healthy foods are lean meats, fish, low-fat dairy, and beans.

4. Load up on antioxidants. These are the nutrients that repair daily damage to your arteries. Fruits and vegetables contain antioxidants. Green tea is another source of antioxidants; it has several powerful antioxidants that reduce cholesterol levels.

5. Cut back on fats. Reduce trans fats from margarine and avoid saturated fats, which are fats that turn solid at room temperature such as butter, cheese, and animal fats. Use olive oil as a substitute for butter or margarine and make sure you buy cold-pressed extra virgin oil as it has more of the healthy antioxidants.

6. Support with supplements. Pick antioxidant vitamin supplements such as Vitamin E and B vitamins, including B6 and folic acid. Add healthy omega-3 fats to your diet by sprinkling a couple of tablespoons of pre-ground flaxseed to your salad, smoothies, or cereal. Flaxseed oil, like fish oil, has been shown in studies to reduce certain cardiac risk factors.

7. Get regular check-ups. Consult with your doctor, but also broaden your choices by seeking advice from natural therapy providers such as a naturopath or nutritionist. No one knows it all, and you must take

responsibility for your own health. Conduct research and catch up on the latest reading.

8. Get good quality sleep. When we sleep, we give the body time and space to carry out the repair work to heal and to boost good health. Insufficient sleep is linked to weight gain, high blood pressure, and other heart disease risk factors. Sufficient sleep is defined as between seven to nine hours.

BOOST HEALING BY CREATING A HEALING ENVIRONMENT

Reducing stress is a major ingredient in the recipe for good health, so find ways to relieve stress in your life. Rethink a tendency to overwork in the office and sort out your priorities so you do not get too upset when work is frustrating. Build support groups and nurture strong relationships. Emotional support from friends and family are stress buffers.

Stack up on stress management tools. There are so many relaxation techniques available to any of us, such as yoga, Tai Chi, Qigong, acupuncture, or guided meditations. Yoga has become commonplace with many community centers offering classes. Acupuncture is recommended as a natural remedy to rebalance the body's energy flow, improve circulation, and blood flow to the heart.

Meditation has been shown to lower cholesterol and reverse any thickening of the carotid arteries. You can join meditation groups, download soothing music, and even find free guided meditations online which you can follow within the sanctuary of your own home. The idea is to have fun and experiment to see which one resonates best with you. Be committed and consistent with the relaxation techniques of your choice; you are making great strides towards better health.

Here's another tip: Do you know how health and beauty spas get you to slow down and chill out by playing slow, meditative music? Notice that they do not have loud rock-and-roll because meditative melodies slow the heart rate, while loud and fast beats rev up our natural heart rate. Prepare a playlist of soft, soothing music to help you take it down a notch.

PAY HEED TO THE MIND-BODY CONNECTION

Health is not just a state of the body, it is also a state of mind. Our bodies react to what we think and how we feel, and the mind-body connection is constantly in play.

It shouldn't surprise you that one of the best mind-body exercises is to have a good laugh. Laughter is the best medicine. We've all heard this before, and it is such a common saying that we often overlook how true the advice is. When you laugh out loud, you can't stay depressed, angry, or frustrated. In fact, a good belly laugh turns these negative emotions on their head.

When you're laughing until your sides hurt, you're doing many good things for your body: You're giving the T-cells a good boost. These are special white blood cells that are crucial to the immune system. They regulate the immune response or directly swoop down on infected cells. The T-cells need to be activated, and a good laugh will do precisely that.

Laughing promotes a sense of well-being. Endorphins are the feel-good chemicals that are produced from exercise. Laughter produces a healthy dose of endorphins and also contributes to an overall positive outlook on life. Those who have a more positive attitude tend to stay healthier or recover faster.

Your body relaxes for up to 45 minutes after laughing. Furthermore, laughter is contagious. Sharing a laugh with someone lowers barriers, promotes intimacy, and enhances relationships, all of which are good things that boost heart health.

Set your mind towards optimal health and successful healing. The change in attitude may seem like a small step, but before you know it, you've made giant strides towards maintaining a healthy heart.

The Greatest Weapon Against Cancer Is Knowledge

Every Cancer Is Different. Learn About Your Risk And Ways to Reduce It

MELANIE R. PALOMARES, M.D., M.S.

Cancer afflicts millions of people and takes hundreds of thousands of lives each year. In 2012, the World Health Organization (WHO) reported 14 million new cancer diagnoses and 8.2 million deaths— and that number is projected to rise in the coming years.[1] Statistics suggest that about 39 percent of men and women will be diagnosed with this disease at some point during their lifetime.[2] The good news is that, today, early

1 World Health Organization Staff, "WHO | Cancer." World Health Organization, 2015. Web. http://www.who.int/mediacentre/factsheets/fs297/en/

2 National Cancer Institute Staff, "SEER Stat Fact Sheets: Cancer of Any Site." National Cancer Institute, 2013. Web. https://seer.cancer.gov/statfacts/html/all.html

detection and specialized treatment for different types of cancer can make all the difference.

Cancer used to be the disease that no one talked about—and, unfortunately, that meant that people at risk didn't even know about their family's medical history. Even today, there's a stigma surrounding cancer patients. In an article for *Cancer World*, the principal periodical of the European School of Oncology, Associate Editor Anna Wagstaff gives a harrowing report of the way societies around the world view cancer:

"Fears that the disease may be infectious can result in people being shunned by friends and neighbours (sic) and excluded from the community. Fears that it is hereditary can ruin the marriage chances of those with a mother or father known to have had cancer. Whole families can find themselves impacted, which can then put intolerable strains on relationships, leaving people with cancer even more isolated."[3]

The good news is that we are far more educated on the matter than we used to be. Today we have a wealth of information available via social media and the internet. The challenge is the quality of information available from such sources, which are not always subject to medical peer review. This has led to more awareness, and there have been more discoveries about lifestyle and environmental risk factors, which may be modified to improve cancer risk.

Studies have shown that the more accurate information one has, the better chance one has to maintain their health. In general, you are far more likely to survive a bout with cancer if you catch it at an early stage. For instance, Mayo Clinic reports the survival rate for colorectal cancer is 90% if it is caught early, although it is the second deadliest cancer in the United States, when all stages

---

3 World Health Organization Staff, "WHO | Cancer." World Health Organization, 2015. Web. http://www. Anna Wagstaff, "Stigma: Breaking the Vicious Cycle." Cancer World, 2013. Web. http://www.cancerworld. org/Articles/Issues/55/July-August-2013/Patient-Voice/602/Stigma-breaking-the-vicious-cycle.html

are considered.[4]

This information may motivate you to pursue cancer screenings, but you should know that those come with their own set of risks. For one thing, screening tests are not 100% reliable. Even when they are conducted by medical professionals you know and trust, the possibility of a false-positive or false-negative result exists. Beyond that, some testing procedures come with their own immediate hazards. Colonoscopies, for example, carry some risk of damaging the lining of the colon.[5] Therefore, it is important to pursue to proper type and frequency of screening for your level of cancer risk.

By far, the best defenses against cancer are prevention and proactivity. The National Cancer Institute estimates that as many as 50-75% of cancer fatalities in the United States are caused by negative lifestyle choices, like smoking, lack of exercise, or poor diet.[6] Just by living a healthy lifestyle, you can reduce your chances of contracting cancer dramatically.

That said, it is most important to know how prone you are to the disease. If the disease runs in your family, or if you think that you may have had an exposure that may increase your risk of developing cancer (examples of such risk factors are discussed throughout this chapter), you need not feel helpless. Your first step is to talk with an oncologist or a general physician with specific training and experience in understanding cancer risk factors to perform an accurate risk assessment. From there, you can obtain personalized cancer screening recommendations tailored to your level of risk. You can also learn about a variety of different precautions that you can take to minimize

---

4 Sharon Theimer, "Mayo Clinic Expert Shares Five Things to Know About Colorectal Cancer." Mayo Clinic News Network, 2016. Web. http://newsnetwork.mayoclinic.org/discussion/mayo-clinic-expert-shares-5-things-to-know-about-colorectal-cancer/

5 National Cancer Institute, "Cancer Screening Overview." National Cancer Institute, 2016. Web. https://www.cancer.gov/about-cancer/screening/patient-screening-overview-pdq

6 National Cancer Institute, NIH, DHHS. Cancer Trends Progress Report – 2011/2012 Update. Bethesda; 2012.

your chances of developing any form of cancer. It all comes down to having a keen knowledge of your personal history and knowing exactly what your body needs at any given time in your life, based on your age and occurrences in your life.

EVALUATING YOUR RISKS

When evaluating and minimizing your risk of developing cancer, it is important to note that one size does not fit all. Each form of cancer comes with a specific and distinct set of risk factors, variables that make you more or less susceptible to cancer development. In general, risk factors for cancer can be filed under two different classifications: genetic and environmental.

Genetic Risk Factors Are Inborn

Those with family histories of cancer, or those who inherit mutated genes from their parents, often have a relatively high chance of developing cancer. By nature, genetic risks are immutable and unalterable; we cannot, after all, change the way we were born. However, it is still important to recognize how your genes affect your chances of developing cancer, so that you may take appropriate preventive measures.

Environmental Risk Factors Are a Product of Nurture

These risk factors revolve around the characteristics of your living area, such as the climate (eg. sun exposure), the quality of the air you breathe, and the food you consume. Unlike genetic factors, environmental factors are, to some extent, subject to change. However, these changes may or may not be within your control, depending on what your living options are and whether you can afford to move.

In general, while there are many types and subtypes of cancer, all associated with different risk factors, screening, treatment, and prevention, in this chapter I will focus on the four most common cancers in the U.S.: breast and gynecologic cancers, colon cancer, lung cancer, and prostate cancer. These "Big Four" account for over 50% of all the cancers that occur in Americans.

BREAST AND GYNECOLOGIC CANCERS

From birth, sex hormones play an instrumental role in your body's growth, maturity and fertility. After you mature, your reproductive health is largely dependent on how well your body maintains the balance between estrogens and androgens. The enzyme aromatase plays a particularly vital part in a woman's reproductive health, breaking down larger hormones in the breasts and ovaries. This is important to note because breast cancer, like most gynecologic cancers, is hormone-driven.

The most important factors in determining breast cancer risk are gender and age. Since breast cancer growth is facilitated by the presence of female hormones, it serves to reason that the illness predominately affects women (but not only women). It also follows that breast cancer is most likely to develop post-maturity, when the body's hormonal activity reaches its peak. This is also the case for most ovarian and uterine cancers. On the other hand, cervical cancer is more likely to occur in young women, particularly those with more sexual activity, though the availability of human papilloma virus (HPV) vaccines will likely change the epidemiology of that disease as they become more commonly used for cancer prevention in girls and young women.

With breast and gynecologic cancers, despite popular belief, the role of inheritance is relatively minor. Although a family history of breast and/or ovarian cancer does make it more likely that you will develop one of these diseases, studies show that less than 15-20% of diagnosed breast cancer patients in America have immediate relatives with the same affliction,[7] and only about 5-10% have a strong family history of breast and/or ovarian cancer associated with a high cancer susceptibility genetic mutation. The most well-known examples are inherited mutations in the BRCA1 or BRCA2 genes, which are associated with the Hereditary Breast and Ovarian Cancer (HBOC) syndrome. Yet other cancer susceptibility genetic mutations, specifically mutations the DNA mismatch repair genes, are associated with a high risk of uterine and ovarian cancer with colon cancer, rather than breast cancer, in an entirely different inheritable entity called Lynch syndrome. In addition, there are gene mutations that carry only an intermediate elevation in risk for developing breast cancer, such as inherited mutations in a gene called PTEN, which are also associated with uterine cancer, thyroid cancer, and colon polyps as part of a less common familial entity called Cowden's syndrome. While there are even a few more familial syndromes that have been described to be associated with breast and/or gynecologic cancer, cervical cancer appears to be related to HPV infection as an environmental risk, with little to no relation to inheritance.

In addition to family history, you should also look into your personal history; breast cancer is more likely to happen in women who had their first period before age 12, as well as those who went through menopause relatively late.[8] The standard use of mammograms for breast cancer screening since the 1980s has shifted this disease to one that is more often caught early, except in younger women who may not have started regular screening yet. Two points

7 breastcancer.org Staff, "U.S. Breast Cancer Statistics." breastcancer.org, 2016. Web. http://www.breastcancer.org/symptoms/understand_bc/statistics
8 Mayo Clinic Staff, "Symptoms and Causes – Breast Cancer." Mayo Clinic, 2016. Web. http://www.mayoclinic.org/diseases-conditions/breast-cancer/symptoms-causes/dxc-20207918

follow from this trend: 1) women who have had findings of changes that occur prior to the development of a full cancer have an opportunity for medical prevention, and 2) it is particularly important to understand a woman's cancer risk in order to adjust screening recommendations to given high-risk women the same opportunity for early detection.

Lastly, diet and physical activity appear to play an important role in the development of these cancers. Obesity has been particularly associated with breast and uterine cancer. In addition, excessive alcohol use has been linked to breast cancer risk, particularly in premenopausal women.

COLORECTAL CANCERS

Colorectal cancers originate in the colon and rectum. The term "colorectal cancer" refers the most common of the cancers that develop within the human digestive tract. Colorectal cancers share a variety of causes and risk factors. One of them is chronic inflammation, as is seen in individuals with a history of the chronic inflammatory bowel diseases (IBD), Crohn's Disease or Ulcerative Colitis. Chronic inflammation can lead to the development of dysplasia, abnormally structured cells in the colon. Dysplastic cells often contain somatic, or non-inherited genetic mutations that are acquired after birth, which have the potential to develop into cancer cells over time.

Also, like breast and ovarian cancers, colorectal cancers have a familial component. In fact, there are some hereditary conditions that increase their carriers' propensity towards colorectal cancer. One such condition is Lynch syndrome, which was mentioned in the previous section, because of its association with uterine and ovarian cancers as well. Another syndrome is called familial adenomatous polyposis (FAP), an inherited condition that causes multiple polyps to grow in the patient's large intestine.[9] There are additional familial syndromes that have been described to be associated with colorectal cancers. These, as well as more detail about other cancer genetics syndromes, may be found at my website, www.caprevinc.org.

Diet is also thought to play a role in colon cancer, with certain elements, such as adequate folate and fiber intake, appearing to take an important role in minimizing risk.[10] Diets that include lots of vegetables, fruits, and whole grains have also been linked with a decreased risk of colon cancer. Dietary fat has been linked to a higher risk of colon cancer, as well as tobacco and alcohol use. The American Institute for Cancer Risk (AICR) estimates that 45% of colon cancers are preventable through diet, staying a healthy weight, and being physically active.[11]

LUNG CANCER

In general, lifestyle and environmental factors play the largest role in the development of lung cancer. This is an important point, in that lung cancer is the most common cause of cancer death in the United States, yet its risk factors are largely modifiable. Thus, it is important to understand these risks so that you can make the best choices for yourself and your family.

While tobacco use is the most well known risk factor, an additional major contributing factor is the exposure to secondhand smoke, or smoke expelled from used cigarettes and tobacco pipes. The American Cancer Society has

---

9 Al-Sukhni W, Aronson M, Gallinger S. "Hereditary colorectal cancer syndromes: familial adenomatous polyposis and lynch syndrome." Surg Clin North Am. 2008 Aug;88(4):819-44, vii. doi: 10.1016/j.suc.2008.04.012.

10 Giovannucci E, Willett WC. "Dietary factors and risk of colon cancer." Ann Med. 1994 Dec;26(6):443-52.

11 http://www.aicr.org/press/press-releases/preventing-colon-cancer-6-steps.html?referrer=https://www.google.com/

shown that secondhand smoke is even more toxic and carcinogenic than the vapor taken in by smokers themselves.[12] Because of this, the risk of lung cancer is relatively high for those who live or work around chronic smokers. Smoking and other tobacco use, such as chewing tobacco, also increases the risk for aerodigestive cancers, such as cancers of the oral cavity, throat, esophagus, and stomach. And because tobacco products can be excreted in the urine, tobacco use is also associated with kidney and bladder cancer.

Another large contributing factor to lung cancer is radon poisoning. Radon is a colorless, odorless substance that spawns from the natural decay of uranium in soil. Commonly, homes, particularly those in suburban or rural areas, can build up large quantities of radon over time as it rises up from the soil and seeps through cracks and flaws in the foundation. This is more common than you might think; in fact, it's responsible for roughly 21,000 lung cancer deaths each year, making it the second largest contributor to lung cancer behind tobacco.[13]

Asbestos is another major environmental factor associated with lung cancer. Asbestos poisoning is associated with a specific kind of lung cancer called mesothelioma. Since the 1980s, several laws have been passed in this country to restrict the availability and usage of asbestos in architecture. In spite of this, we still see a steady number of new mesothelioma diagnoses each year—about 3,000 annually, as estimated by the Mesothelioma Center.[14]

---

12 American Cancer Society, "Health Risks of Secondhand Smoke." ACS, 2015. Web. http://www.cancer.org/cancer/cancercauses/tobaccocancer/secondhand-smoke

13 Janet McCabe, "For peace of mind, add 'test for radon' to your 2016 to-do list." EPA Connect, 2016. Web.https://blog.epa.gov/blog/2016/01/test-for-radon/

14 The Mesothelioma Center, "Mesothelioma - Overview of Malignant Mesothelioma Cancer." asbestos.org, 2016. Web. https://www.asbestos.com/mesothelioma/

PROSTATE CANCER

Prostate cancer is the most common cancer occurring in American men, aside from skin cancer.[15] In 2016 alone, 26,120 American men were reported to have died from this affliction. In fact, one in seven men will be diagnosed with prostate cancer in their lifetime. Like breast and gynecologic cancers, prostate cancer is largely influenced by hormones; the difference, of course, is that it feeds off of androgens, male hormones, rather than estrogens.

Age is also a risk factor. Prostate cancer is seldom diagnosed in men younger than 40, and roughly 60% of cases are diagnosed in men at least 65 years of age.[16] Heredity and genes also play a role in prostate cancer development, although no highly penetrant cancer susceptibility genes have been described to date, unlike with breast, gynecologic, and colorectal cancers. Nevertheless, men who are closely related to prostate cancer patients are twice as likely to develop it themselves. The risk heightens even further if a man has more than one affected relative.

CANCER SCREENING

Cancer screening methods range from physical exam or self-exam to blood tests and specialized x-rays, such as mammograms, or procedures, such as colonoscopies. These methods are recommended to be performed at different frequencies depending upon age, family history, and other risk factors.

Concerns about false positive results, which can lead to unnecessary tests

---

15 Rebecca L. Siegel, Kimberly D. Miller and Ahmedin Jemal, "Cancer Statistics, 2016." CA: A Cancer Journal for Clinicians, 2016. Web. http://onlinelibrary.wiley.com/doi/10.3322/caac.21332/full

16 Prostate Cancer Foundation, "Prostate Cancer FAQs." Web. http://www.pcf.org/site/c.leJRIROrEpH/b.5800851/k.645A/Prostate_Cancer_FAQs.htm

and patient anxiety, as well as to overdiagnosis and overtreatment, has led to widespread controversy regarding different screening techniques. In addition, due to concerns about health care costs, cancer screening policies differ from country to country. This is why different guidelines are often offered by different medical organizations, which unfortunately leads to confusion for both consumers and health care professionals.

It is for this reason that I highly recommend seeking the advice of a physician with specific training and experience in understanding cancer risk factors to perform an accurate risk assessment. From there, you can obtain personalized recommendations specified to your risk level. Resources for determining your general category of cancer risk and, if appropriate, how to find a referral to a qualified health care professional near you can be found at my website, www.caprevinc.org. Webinars on this topic are in development and will be available at that site as well.

REDUCING YOUR RISK

While cancer screening can help with early detection of cancer, which does improve outcomes with cancer treatment, as mentioned earlier in this chapter, it is important to remember that you have the power to help mitigate your chances of developing cancer in the first place (or getting it again, if you are a cancer survivor). Fighting the disease is a matter of recognizing what you can and cannot control, and focusing on what you can control. Your personal choices on a day-to-day basis can make a huge difference in your personal war against cancer, and you cannot go into battle without knowing what the consequences of those choices are.

LIFESTYLE INTERVENTIONS

A balanced, careful diet is key to fighting cancer. The influence of your food intake on your cancer risk cannot be overstated. Some foods actually have the potential to increase your risk of developing cancer, so it's vital to know what to eat, what to abstain from, and what to limit.

Diet: Plant-Based Foods

When it comes to prevention of and survivorship with cancer, fruits, vegetables and whole grains are the most desirable foods you can eat. Cancer.net educates patients about the link between excessive body fat and the development of several types of cancer, including the aforementioned colorectal cancer.[17] As such, your best bet is to eat foods that are low in fat and high in fiber. Plant-based food groups (vegetables, fruits, nuts, whole grains and legumes) all fit the bill. Fiber-rich foods in particular will help you along the way. Fiber is the broom of the digestive system, sweeping your intestines clean and keeping your digestive processes running at regular intervals. Because of this, fiber helps flush carcinogenic compounds out of your body, thus preventing cancer from growing.

Diet: Animal Products

While a plant-based diet is wholly important to cancer prevention, this does not mean you have to swear off meat and dairy altogether. You should, however, place significant limits on how much animal-based food you take in. Most people, especially Americans, consume far more meat than they should.

---

17 Cancer.net Editorial Board, "Obesity, Weight and Cancer Risk." Cancer.net, 2016. Web. http://www.cancer.net/navigating-cancer-care/prevention-and-healthy-living/obesity-and-cancer/obesity-weight-and-cancer-risk

In general, meat should not constitute more than a small fraction of the calories you take in per day. It's also important to recognize that some meats are better than others. Poultry and fish, for instance, are leaner and healthier alternatives to beef and pork. It's also a good idea to stay away from processed meats, like hot dogs and salami.

Physical Activity

Get moving! Exercise, particularly aerobic exercise, is an integral part of weight management, and by extension, cancer prevention. It is possible to reduce your risk for colorectal and breast cancer in particular with a regular exercise regimen. The AICR recommends sustained physical activity for at least 30 minutes a day.[18]

In addition to avoidance of obesity, which has been linked to an increasing number of different cancer types,[19] there are other benefits provided by regular exercise. For one thing, it keeps your metabolism running quickly and efficiently, which in turn will keep your weight at a healthy level. It also serves to strengthen your immune system, which plays an integral role in your body's defenses against cancer. Finally, regular exercise helps regulate your hormone levels which, as mentioned before, play a key role in the development of gynecologic cancers.

Stress Management

---

18 American Institute for Cancer Research, "Physical Activity Recommended for Preventing Cancer." AICR, 2016. Web. http://www.aicr.org/reduce-your-cancer-risk/recommendations-for-cancer-prevention/recommendations_02_activity.html

19 Béatrice Lauby-Secretan, Ph.D., Chiara Scoccianti, Ph.D., Dana Loomis, Ph.D., Yann Grosse, Ph.D., Franca Bianchini, Ph.D., and Kurt Straif, M.P.H., M.D., Ph.D., for the International Agency for Research on Cancer Handbook Working Group. Body Fatness and Cancer — Viewpoint of the IARC Working Group. N Engl J Med 2016; 375:794-798, August 25, 2016.

Chronic stress can affect body system functioning, particularly the immune system, and a weak immune system makes the body a more hospitable environment for cancer cells to grow. Stress also leads to release of a hormone called cortisol, which leads to truncal obesity, thereby leading to an increased risk of obesity-related cancers. Cortisol, along with other stress-related chemicals called catecholamines, has also been shown to directly facilitate cancer growth. Yet other stress hormones can inhibit a process called anoikis, which normally kills diseased cells and prevents them from spreading. Finally, chronic stress leads to increased production of growth factors that promote inflammation and new blood supply, which could potentially feed a developing cancer, as well as provide an environment for invasion and metastasis, or spread.[20]

While it is not realistic to avoid all sources of stress in our lives, it is possible to manage our relationship to external stressors. Mindfulness practices, such as meditation and yoga, can be very helpful in this regard. Getting adequate sleep not only supports successful stress management, but also allows to body to get the rest it needs to function well. Reading personal development books can help define knowledge and skills on how to manage situations that may be new or uncomfortable to us. Seeking the support of a mental health professional can be very helpful in identifying healthy ways to manage stress specific to your situation.

MEDICATIONS

If you are particularly worried about your susceptibility to cancer, there are a variety of cancer-suppressing medications that you can use. While some of them can be particularly potent cancer deterrents, they can be dangerous if

---

20 Myrthala Moreno-Smith, Susan K Lutgendorf, and Anil K Sood, Impact of stress on cancer metastasis. Future Oncol. 2010 Dec; 6(12): 1863–1881.

used improperly. As with any drug, consult your physician before taking any of these medications, and be sure that you know about all of the side effects and potential risks.

For those with family histories of colon cancer, the Food and Drug Administration (FDA) recommends Celecoxib, most often known under the brand name 'Celebrex.' It works by disrupting the formation of polyps in your digestive tract, thus preventing cancer cells from growing there. However, those with histories of heart problems should be wary of using Celebrex. It is classified as a Non-Steroidal Anti-Inflammatory Drug (NSAID), and some NSAIDs can heighten your risk of heart disease and stroke.[21] In some patients, it may also cause serious gastrointestinal problems, including stomach ulcers.[22] Some studies suggest that aspirin may be an alternative for colon cancer risk reduction.

For breast cancer, there is a class of drugs known as selective estrogen response modifiers, or SERMs for short. In general, they have two primary functions; firstly, they are designed to suppress the production of estrogen in certain body tissues, particularly those in the breast. Secondly, they take on the functions that estrogen would normally fulfill, thus enabling your body to function properly without facilitating breast cancer growth.

But, like NSAIDs, SERMs have their own set of risks. Tamoxifen, for instance, heightens your risk of developing blood clots and having a stroke (though this risk is still relatively small). Tamoxifen can also exacerbate the symptoms of menopause, including hot flashes and vaginal dryness.[23] Tamoxifen has been shown to slightly increase the risk of uterine cancer, but for women who have a high risk for developing breast cancer, this risk is

---

21 The Internet Drug Index, "Celebrex." RxList, 2011. Web. http://www.rxlist.com/celebrex-drug.htm
22 Omudhome Ogbru, "Celebrex Side Effects Center." RxList, 2016. Web. http://www.rxlist.com/celebrex-side-effects-drug-center.htm
23 National Cancer Institute, "Hormone Therapy for Breast Cancer." 2012. Web. http://www.cancer.gov/cancertopics/factsheet/Therapy/hormone-therapy-breast

outweighed by its breast cancer reduction effects.

For postmenopausal women, an aromatase inhibitor called exemestane (brand name: Aromasin) is another alternative for medical breast cancer risk reduction. This drug may also be associated with menopausal symptoms, and also is associated with bone loss and thus may not be a good option for women with osteoporosis or osteopenia.

Prostate cancer patients have their own class of hormonal suppressant preventive agents, called 5α-reductase inhibitors. Two medications fall into this class of drugs, finasteride (brand name: Proscar) and dutasteride (Avodart). Similar to SERMs, they work by suppressing the production of androgens in the patient's body, thus preventing a cancer from growing. But, just like SERMS, these drugs may come with side effects.

Despite their side effects, these medications can be very useful for individuals with a high risk for a specific cancer, which underscores the importance of talking with your doctor about cancer risk assessment. If you are found to be at high risk, a cancer prevention specialist may offer you consultation to see if the benefits of a particular drug far outweigh its side effects in your particular case.

SURGICAL INTERVENTION

Preventive surgery is a last resort, as it can be stressful, risky and exceedingly expensive. It should only be used if your risk of developing cancer is high enough to justify it.

The most common form of preventive surgery is a bilateral mastectomy, the removal of one or both of your breasts. A mastectomy is often used to remove cancerous tissue in the breast, but it can also be used proactively to prevent the growth of cancer in that area. While a mastectomy will reduce the risk of breast cancer by a huge margin, it will not eliminate the risk altogether. Also, as you would expect, there are a variety of unrelated risks that come with the mastectomy procedure. Like any surgery, a mastectomy can lead to scarring, disfigurement, infection in the surgical area and blood clots. As such, only patients with an exceedingly high susceptibility to breast cancer should consider this option.

Similarly, prophylactic bilateral salpingo-oophorectomy (removal of both fallopian tubes and ovaries to prevent ovarian cancer) or prophylactic colectomy (removal of all or part of the colon to prevent colon cancer) may be considered in special high-risk patients.

These are just a few of the methods you can use to snuff out cancer before it grows. In short, the best way to minimize your chance of developing cancer is to take care of yourself. Have a keen awareness of what your body needs on a day-to-day basis, and act accordingly. Watch what you eat, keep track of your physical activity, and consult an experienced physician. If you'd like to learn more about the various types of cancer and what you can do to lower your own risk, please visit www.caprevinc.org or call 844-PREV-INC.

In summary, reducing your risk of getting cancer is possible. Start by understanding your family medical history as well as lifestyle and environmental risk factors. Have a positive attitude, a strict sense of self-awareness, and the willingness to change what you can and accept what you can't but with a proactive plan to manage your risk.

If you would like to know more about Dr. Melanie R. Palomares, M.D., M.S., and Cancer Prevention, Inc. please visit http://www.caprevinc.org/.

Break Free From Your Pain Cycle

Winning the Battle and Conquering Autoimmune Disease

SEEMA GIRI

"It is not a journey of understanding; it is a journey of trust. It is a journey of surrendering every aspect of your soul over to the light."

— Panache Desai

D o you have an autoimmune disease? Did you suffer for years before obtaining a diagnosis? Have you been told there's no cure for your condition? If so, I suggest you look beyond your doctors and dive into the ocean of information that's available today regarding autoimmune conditions. You can also begin your journey back to health, take charge of your recovery by reading this chapter. That's right, I know you can reclaim your life. I've done it, and so can you!

"Sometimes it's controversy; but we all have choices that we make."
— **Solomon Burke**

There's a rising healthcare epidemic today. According to the American Autoimmune Related Diseases Association (AARDA), nearly 50 million Americans have some form of an autoimmune disorder. Business Wire, a Berkshire Hathaway company, has reported, "The global autoimmune diseases treatment market is estimated to grow at a [Compound Annual Growth Rate] CAGR of 3.80 for the forecasted period, and its market value is expected to reach $45.54 billion by 2022, up from $36.41 billion in 2016." Also, the National Institute of Health (NIH) claims that annual direct health care costs for autoimmune diseases are in the range of $100 billion (source: NIH presentation by Dr. Fauci, NIAID). According to the data published by the NIH, autoimmune disorders have been ranked in the top ten types of disorders leading to increasing mortality rates amongst women. These numbers are alarming!

As if this isn't enough, there's evidence today that the government, as well as agriculture and pharmaceutical companies, have been creating controversial dietary guidelines that primarily serve their needs rather than the needs of the people. This has been reported by major news channels, the Huffington Post and Marion Nestle, the consumer activist, nutritionist and academic who specializes in the politics of food and dietary choice. Roberto Ferdman of the Washington Post discusses this concern at length in his exposé "We Don't Know What to Eat." It gets worse. Soda companies are funding 96 health groups in the US—as covered by Time Magazine on Oct. 10, 2016. There's also evidence of an increasing number of illnesses nationally, globally and even in our children today.

So let me ask you, are we really getting objective information for our highest good? I certainly don't think so and it breaks my heart to see how little our lives are valued. What's the difference between lab rats and us? It's not as bad as it could be because there are an equal number of medical doctors, lobbyists, alternative medical practitioners and eastern holistic practitioners doing research and presenting their results. The recent movie "Heal" is a film by Kelly Noonan Gores about the power of the mind to heal the body, featuring Deepak Chopra, Bruce Lipton and Marianne Williamson. The film "Autoimmune Secrets" by Jonathan Otto also comes to mind. Then there's me taking responsibility to share my journey as a member of the global community.

"There are two primary choices in life: to accept conditions as they exist, or accept the responsibility for changing them."
— Denis Waitley

The good news is that you and your family don't have to be part of the statistics just mentioned. And you don't have to be affected by propaganda. You simply need to accept responsibility for changing your life and not accept anyone giving you limited information. This is more critical today than ever before.

It's important to make the CHOICE to take control of your health and that of your family. The answer isn't more medication. The answer is becoming more aware and educated. The answer lies in identifying the root cause. I'm passionate about educating you on this topic because life is a collection of precious, irreplaceable moments. Mothers should witness every moment of their children's lives. Children should not be robbed of their childhood. Fathers and husbands should not have to watch their family struggle and feel helpless. Families should not have to go thru the trauma of strained relationships because of lack of trust and differing beliefs. My family and I have lived through this. In Maya Angelou's words, "My mission in life is to not merely survive, but to thrive; and to do so with some passion, some compassion, some humor and some style"

"Our lives begin to end the day we become silent about things that matter."
— **Martin Luther King Jr.**

Will you join me in creating a revolution to break free from your pain cycle? I hope so. I'm going to share some of my story with you, and then outline the changes you'll need to make on your journey back to health, as well as some resources to help you.

"We are all Working Together; that's the Secret."
— Sam Walton

There's a quiet but pervasive problem in the world today. It's a sense of shame resulting from mental and physical health conditions. People feel they can't speak out, that others won't understand—and they're right! This is impacting families; it's impacting men, women and children (who are going to be the leaders of tomorrow). The problem can also be seen as a race to keep up with the acceptable norms of social and economic standards or as we say, "keeping up with the Jones'." Technology has helped increase anxiety with the ease of reach and exposure at the click of a button.

My focus in this chapter is going to be mainly on women in the middle class. Why women? Out of the 50 million Americans that have autoimmune disease 80 percent are women. I believe this is so because we are part of the sandwich generation; we need to take care of elderly parents and children. This leads to compromises in our own health. There just isn't enough time. And, of course, there are the effects of hormonal imbalances. Also, women are the primary caregivers in the family. They're at the centre of the family and have a great influence on everyone else. If we help the women—who are the counselors, the ones who spend the most time with our kids, and to who others constantly come to share their confidences— and they become whole people, what do think will happen to those around them? They're going to change.

Today, the majority of health issues are due to chronic stress, environmental toxicity and chemical toxicity. Our food is genetically modified and our soil is depleted of the essential nutrients. We aren't getting nutrient dense food. And don't forget emotional and mental toxicities. We don't realize the impact of these on our health. My own autoimmune story has primarily arisen from emotional toxicities and food, as you will see as I unfold my experience.

I'll even speak directly to the Indian community. Why? Because as a culture we keep our feelings to ourselves and internalize things quite a bit. The next epidemic is already here and it's psychological in nature. The stress women experience these days is phenomenal. This can be seen throughout society as a whole via school shootings and hate crimes. Resolving these issues requires getting back to basics. We need to slow down, breathe and listen to each other. We need to be authentic, open our hearts and share our issues. The more we reach out to our community, the easier it will be to support each other in coming up with solutions. Once this is done, you can have sustainable energy and health to be able to enjoy what you love to do as a professional or an entrepreneur.

Visit www.seemagiri.com for a free guide on: How to Reduce Stress.

With an autoimmune disease you tend to forget what normal is. There are layers of pain, layers of suppressed and unprocessed emotions—you know, the ones you say are ok but that still bother you in the back of your mind and that limit your life. To reclaim your health, you have to go through these layers, like you would an onion, and you have to reset and recharge at every step. Each layer brings a new insight and wisdom. While you may never return to the "normal" you used to know, you can absolutely create a new normal that is even better than before. This is like keeping your computer running efficiently; you have to begin deleting files that are no longer serving you and clean your hard drive. In the same way, from time to time you need to release your pent up feelings and resentments and allow forgiveness for others and yourself.

"Forgiveness doesn't excuse anyone's actions. Forgiveness stops actions from destroying your heart."
— **Karen Salmansohn**

You need to give yourself permission to let go of hurtful experiences and a painful past. This comes from acknowledging your situation rather than living in denial; taking responsibility and making the change. Master Choa Kok Sui, Founder of Modern Pranic Healing and Arhatic Yoga, states inner forgiveness deals with love and compassion, while outer forgiveness deals with the necessity to create order and justice. While you can forgive internally, the individual still must deal with consequences or punishment. For example, when a child steals for the first time, you can forgive them but still give age appropriate punishment so he or she doesn't steal again. These two types of forgiveness must be balanced, all while coming from a place of love for yourself and the other person. Otherwise the dis-ease manifests into disease.

"The journey of a thousand miles begins with one single step."
— **Lao Tzu**

I lived a life of confinement, isolation and depression for more than 20 years. I was misdiagnosed by multiple doctors for several years with anxiety, depression, stress, chronic fatigue syndrome, psychological issues and was even called a hypochondriac when the test results showed up normal each time. The worst part was that I had started to believe the pain, inflammation and lack of energy were all in my head. Even my family agreed with my doctors, saying that I needed to just get over it; I wasn't the only one in the world who had health issues, and I needed to learn to deal with it better and move on. Eventually, I was on over 26 medications, many of them causing additional side effects. Not a single bottle came with a warning that said, "may cause extreme sexiness" but rather, came with labels that said, "may cause dizziness, heart problems, depression, suicidal thoughts, etc." Many times I felt the side effects were more dangerous than my actual health problems.

The biggest problem with autoimmune disease is that you look perfectly healthy from the outside while you are having a tsunami on the inside that never ends. Life becomes limited to home and doctor visits, but people don't understand why. Secondly, it mimics many diseases that express themselves with lethargy, fatigue, dizziness, sleeplessness and inflammation. Doctors have to rule out numerous options. I was devastated and felt pushed into a corner. I was a burden on my family. The battle had taken so many years I could understand their frustration as caregivers. And even though there was a dim little voice in my head continuously saying there had to be a better way and that I was meant to have a better life, I fell into a deeper depression. I wasn't being heard by anyone and felt the best way to end everyone's misery was to end the problem, me. I had reached my breaking point and attempted suicide. That's how helpless and hopeless I felt. My thinking was that at least then my family could live a life without limits.

Following the suicide attempt, my family started to take me more seriously, particularly my husband, Upendra. I also realized that I did have a larger purpose in life, that I was meant to make a profound contribution to the world. Yet, there was still doubt in my heart. My greatest strengths were perseverance and courage. I had to use these attributes to fight for a life of possibilities and take charge of my recovery. I chose to listen to that tiny voice that said I was meant to have a better life and continued on my quest until I found a young doctor who believed me, took the time to actively listen to me, and finally did some new tests that enabled him to diagnose me with fibromyalgia and rheumatoid arthritis. Hypothyroidism was diagnosed earlier.

My journey to a "new normal" taught me many things. For example, I realized that the doctors were experimenting with different protocols. This knowledge prompted me to do my own experiments, even though my doctors had told me that lifestyle changes wouldn't make any difference to my condition. I had to try. I was encouraged to find that every time I made a decision, the universe always provided the right resources in terms of people and tools.

I first started making changes to my lifestyle with the help of my friend Mrs. Veena Singla, who introduced me to a whole food nutritional supplement, then exercise and personal development. I could tell I was progressing forward, but then I would go two steps backward, sometimes ten. However, I was persistent and consistent in my efforts to get well.

Because I had lost so much precious time, I hired several coaches to achieve my goals faster—the best investment I ever made in myself. Through their tested systems, life experiences and the perfect balance of empathy, ability to show me my blind spots, and not allowing me to hide, I got unbelievable results quickly. As I continued my journey, working with various therapists, counselors and coaches, I realized how many suppressed and unprocessed emotions I had bottled up inside. These were tough and scary to get through. It took several years of processing and removing layer after layer of emotion, but I managed to get closer to the core of the onion. There were some key pivotal moments that really impacted my life, but I kept peeling away those layers, one at a time.

"We didn't realize we were making memories, we just knew we were having fun."
— **Winnie The Pooh**

My problems began early in life. My parents were strict. They focused on excellence and were always setting new benchmarks (it was more like a sliding benchmark), that made me feel I could never reach their high standards and which led me to believe I wasn't good enough. My parents' constant pressure changed my basic nature, and I became a quiet introvert who kept to myself. You see, I was a naturally outgoing child who was unafraid of strangers (I loved to go on adventures and talk to all the people I would meet). But my behaviour scared my parents. Being in a country where language was a barrier and in a culture we didn't really understand, there were barriers my parents saw that I didn't see. To me, the locals were just people with a different skin color and language. My parents, however, felt I would be safer if I was quiet and controlled. I was disciplined constantly. I used to get a lot of punishments—from scolding to being grounded to taking away my partner in crime, my bike. This is when I discovered the bus. I started taking the bus to different parts of Berlin, the city in Germany where I lived. There would be times I would even come home at 10 or 11 p.m. I know, I know a seven-year-old should not come home so late, but it didn't phase me, as soon as my punishment was up I would do the same thing. I was hungry for adventures and expeditions! I could not stay in the box and have a life with limits.

Even in India, my playmates weren't limited to children but included monkeys, goats and cows. I was born in Shimla, India, a small town located in the middle ranges of the Himalayas. It's the capital city of Himachal Pradesh. Shimla is a lovely hill station that was the summer capital during the British ruling. I spent a considerable amount of time in the village with my grandparents where I had unlimited time to play. I've had a cow ram its horn into my stomach and pin me against the side of the house. I was bitten by a monkey. And I would hang the kids (baby goats) in the branches of our tree and leave them there (don't worry someone would get them down). This used to be all in a day's work. Now that I have children myself, I realize that I was a handful. My children really had a hard time in getting away with many things. My son, Aman, was equally as determined and managed to challenge me.

There are other significant traumas that have impacted my health, some from which I am still healing and find difficult to talk about. These unpleasant experiences led me to believe that due to the color of my skin and being a girl I wasn't good enough and should be invisible. At one point I was beaten so badly that I almost fainted and was covered in blood. I was also accused of stealing a pencil box, where the teacher pinned me against the wall and screamed in my face. These things happened in Owings Mills, MD, where I was the only Indian in the class. Then in Amherst, MA, when

I was ten years old, I endured the most traumatic experience in my life, one that would shape the rest of my future. It left me numb and speechless. I felt that the ground I was standing on was pulled from underneath me. I had nowhere to turn, no one to talk to, no one to believe me. I went thru life like a zombie. I wouldn't even feel the burn of scalding tea on my hand. I believed that I deserved bad things to happen to me.

I became secluded and was a total introvert, limiting my life to only school and home. I internalized a lot of my feelings. My parents couldn't really understand what I was going through. Sometimes I attempted to share my feelings, but I was told I was not supposed to feel that way and to study harder. My parents were working very hard to make a good living and provide a good life for us. They were also supporting my grandparents and my father's younger brother in India. My mother also started working retail on weekends. So that made me the babysitter for my two younger brothers. I didn't want to add to their stress.

About the time we moved to Germany I began the unexplainable manifesting of swollen hands and arms. Then a problem with my hip put me in the hospital for a month. They couldn't explain the issue. Again, we did the medical dance with the doctors: x-rays, tests, etc., with no logical explanations.

At first, I lived a double life. I had to be one way at home in front of my parents and another way at school to try to be accepted. At home I was quiet and invisible. At school I was more extroverted. But, eventually, I succumbed and lost connection to myself. I finally opened the box myself, stepped into it, sat down and closed the flaps. I lived life within the prescribed limit. If I liked the kind of things my father did, then life was easy. If it was anything outside of his wishes, it wasn't allowed. He had a certain idea of how he wanted life, family and kids to be. It was our job to fit in.

Over the years my health continued to be problematic, and I would see a series of doctors. They would do the same tests that would produce normal results. By the time I was in my 20's and married, I was sleeping 16 to 17 hours per day, and when I did get up, I felt like I had been hit by a transport truck. I was going from doctor to doctor to doctor, and it got to the point where I couldn't do the one-hour commute to and from work. I would fall asleep anywhere, even while driving. Now I was really beginning to think that I wasn't human. How can one have so many health issues/incidents without any explanations? I went wild in my imagination with the possibilities. The doctors were able to identify hypothyroidism fairly quickly. When I found out that there really was something tangibly wrong with me, I broke down in the doctor's office and cried. Six months later I was back in the same office because I was still having inflammation and pain. By now I was seeing Dr. Rusk at University of Pennsylvania. He was the first doctor who believed me, and who said my pain was real (that was another hug the doctor, crying moment) and sent me to an endocrinologist who confirmed, after a series of new tests, that I had fibromyalgia and the onset of rheumatoid arthritis. That was another joyous moment in my life. My pain finally had a name. Wow! Now I can be cured! I thought. Then came the shock. They told me there is no cure, just medications to help me manage the symptoms, and that as I age I may even become disabled. I felt like I was standing in court with a judge giving me a sentence: "You are hereby sentenced to a life of pain, misery and heartache. You'll be on medication for the rest of your life. You'll forever be dependent on others as well as a burden. Your life without limits has come to an end!" They told me to exercise—which was a catch 22. I was often in so much pain that it was impossible to exercise, and when I did exercise, I hurt more.

One day my doctor suggested that if I was considering pregnancy, I might find some relief there, as statistics showed that people like me often had permanent change after pregnancy. I wasn't considering pregnancy, but during this time we had a close family friend who had these two adorable kids, Mohit and Arjun. They were loving and authentic. The giving and receiving of unconditional love was amazing. The children were with me so much that people began to think they were mine, which finally got me considering to have my own. When I decided to go ahead, pregnancy was wonderful. I had no pain, my inflammation went away and I lost weight. I had never been happier and I even felt beautiful, something I had never experienced before.

Childbirth was tough though. I ended up having 40 hours of labour. I had preeclampsia, so they had to induce me. I eventually went through an emergency C-Section. However, for the first month everything was great. I couldn't believe I could love anyone so much as I did my son Aman. Then, I started to have symptoms of inflammation and pain to the point that I was bedridden for several months. I was so inflamed I couldn't even hold my baby. I couldn't do anything. There were times when my husband would just put him on the bed beside me so I could feel him and look at him. I couldn't do anything more than that. I finally said this is ridiculous; this is not the way I want to live. I decided I needed to be free from this torment. That was the beginning of my recovery.

So, here is what I learned… When you have a decision to make, always decide without worrying about the how. This is where courage comes into play. You see, in speaking to numerous people in chronic pain I've found they're so used to having a predictable life with support that they begin to enjoy the constant sympathy and attention they receive. As a result, they don't want to change; they're afraid they won't get the same type of love and attention once they are better. I had the same kind of feelings as all the others, but I took the chance anyway. I knew the life of appreciation and courage was far better than sympathy. I've never regretted it. And, now, I'm being recognized for taking action.

At first, it was just Upendra and I. We had family, but they lived far away. My mother had come for two weeks right after I had my baby, but that was it. Upendra was also quite amazing. He was my rock. He would prepare meals for my son and me before going to work, putting the food by my side within reach. I would have to start getting up 45 minutes prior to Aman's feeding. Yes, it would take me 45 minutes of pain, agony and tears to sit up to feed him. I had limited mobility. Upendra would come home and get back to cooking and cleaning. He wouldn't get much time to rest but he never complained or got upset. He was always very optimistic and looked ahead to the future. I guess it was easier for him than for me since he's a visionary guy. Which is why I didn't understand when he started to agree with the doctors that maybe the pain was in my head. Now that I think about it, we had an arranged marriage and had only been married for two years, so he didn't get the chance to know who I really was. We were a work in progress. With all my tests coming back as normal, I guess I would feel that way too. At that time though, I was furious that this thought could even come into his mind.

"The greatest gift of life is friendship, and I have received it."
— **Hubert H. Humphrey**

It was at this time that a close family friend, Mrs. Veena Singla, came on the scene. She was someone who really cared for me regardless of how busy she was with her own family. She also had experience with whole food nutrition. While growing up in India, her family grew their own food, so she had experienced the benefits of farm-to-table concepts, such as fresh fruits and vegetables. She was familiar with the Standard American Diet (SAD) and was also a cancer detection specialist, so she understood the science. In her research for better alternative supplements she'd come across a whole food supplement called Juice Plus. She ordered me to start taking it. I did so because I trusted her, and she was taking it too. However, it was the catalyst the nutritional base, for me to start taking responsibility for my own health. It helped reduce the inflammation and the pain. I was also able to get up and—within four months—start taking care of myself and my baby. This enabled me to make healthier choices. I ate less processed food, did a lot of research and went to a lot of seminars. This opened me up to a whole new community that believed in alternative methods and brought me into contact with people who had similar experiences, confirming to me that it was not all in my head, and that I wasn't crazy. I can't tell you what a relief this was to me. This is when I started to trust myself again. I started to believe that I could live a life without limits. I began to eat less meat and got off wheat, dairy, sugar and processed foods. I was able to exercise on a regular basis, and started working on my mindset.

"When I break the pattern, I break ground. I rebuild when I break down. I wake up more awake than I've been before."
— **Pluto**

The internal light and the constant voice declaring, "there has to be something better for me" and, "I am meant for so much more" was strong enough that I was able to break the pattern of my behaviour. Today I feel that my son, Aman, was the angel who came to me to make me take the steps I did. You see, doing anything for myself was very difficult. Indian culture is such that the focus is more outward. You are to be giving and caring for members of the family, rather than for yourself. I followed what my mom and grandmother did. I felt caring for my needs was being selfish. I think many women around the globe have felt the same way. Had it not been for the needs of my son, who was born in January of 1998, I wouldn't have taken that first step. I am in gratitude to God and my son for this.

I continued on with my healing journey and found women circles that supported my quest. I noticed a pattern that no matter where I went I always had one or two authentic friends who were there to support me. Whether it was to talk, help with the kids or embark on a girl's night out.

The integration of all of The Four Pillars of Health (nutrition, exercise, mindset and spirituality) has helped me be pain free. On April 27, 2000 when I held my daughter Ashima (my second angel) in my arms for the first time, I wanted her to not be burdened with the generational limitations and beliefs that I had. In order for that to happen I had to change and live differently. This meant overcoming the fears and beliefs I'd carried for several years. It meant breaking the pattern. Ashima inspired me to go even deeper. I wanted our background, culture and challenges to empower my children, to be their strength and foundation. I wanted them to be proud of their 5,000-year heritage. Aman and Ashima have also been great teachers to me. They taught me what unconditional love is. They showed me that they will love me for who I am, even if I don't do anything for them. As I've mentioned, I was taught by my parents that if I didn't do certain things, like getting good grades, then other things would be taken away from me. I was doing the same to my children, I would measure their love by how well they listened to me, but I think they must be old souls because they let me know it didn't have to be that way. You don't have to have one or the other; it's not "or" but "and." Imagine! Loving me just for me! That day I could feel years of built-up walls of shame and heaviness that I had carried all that time melt away. It felt like I lost 30 pounds that day.

It took a long time, but I finally realized all you have to do is begin to care for yourself. You need to show others how to love you by providing them an example through self-love. So often, you do everything for your loved ones, in the hope they'll return the same. But if you don't care for yourself first they'll have no idea as to what you really need in return. Could it be this easy?

By this time, I was hooked on Oprah's "SuperSoul Sunday." I had read several spiritual books by Ekart Tolle, Brene Brown, Elizabeth Lesser and learned how to live a conscious life where you make deliberate choices based on your values and your truth. In doing so, I finally learned that you must be courageous enough to take the first step towards change. As you do this you increase your energetic vibration level and attract like things. As you live better, your vibration increases and you attract similar things within the same vibration level. This is where the saying comes in, "change your thoughts, change your life." For example, those who always think negatively have negative things continue to happen to them. Similarly, those who always think positive, or are optimistic, have more positive things happen to them.

It was with these realizations that I noticed I was attracting more positive, accomplished and heart-centered women who took better care of themselves and their families and were pursuing their passions. I also noticed that I began to release people—even family members—who didn't support me, who were full of negative energy and who drained me of life. I learned that in order to change your life you must be prepared to change the five people you keep company with regularly. You'll find it makes a dramatic difference.

"When people walk away from you, let them go. Your destiny is never tied to anyone who leaves you, and it doesn't mean they are bad people. It just means that their part in your story is over."
— Tony McCollum

I started to believe in myself, that I was worthy, and I deserve the best.

"A woman who is convinced that she deserves to accept only the best challenges herself to give the best. Then she is living phenomenally."
— **Maya Angelou**

In 2003 we had the opportunity to go to India. We thought we would go for six months to see if the kids and I would be able to adjust to it. I was excited. I'd always wanted to live in India as an adult, and it was a great time for our kids to get to know our family and culture. Upendra has a big family: six brothers, their spouses, their kids and his extended family. This was scary because I didn't have any close friends or family there. This was an opportunity for us to not only serve our country and the people but also to reconnect with ourselves. Project management was our vehicle to do so. We built our company to 250 employees and trained nearly 100,000 people on project, program and portfolio management. While managing the operation, I trained and counseled professionals on which project management certification would be right for them, based on their years of experience and ambition. I started seeing a pattern of health challenges they were experiencing due to project deadlines and the odd hours required to support global operations. Many had shared that the reason for being in a company or a particular job wasn't because of their passion but because of need. I saw this as a global issue, not just in India. I believe a seed was planted, and I would often think about how I could contribute to people by helping them become healthier and living more fulfilling lives.

As I got to know my in-laws better, I developed a special relationship with my mother-in-law and one particular sister-in-law. Despite the vast differences of our upbringing, my mother-in-law and I connected deeply. She loved me like a son, calling me her seventh son. This is the highest honor she could give me. My sister-in-law's name is Nischal Di. How close are we? Even our birthdays are just a day apart! Nischal Di showed me the parts of myself I'd forgotten. On a regular basis, she would point out my strengths. In all these years, she was the first person who focused on that. She even stood up to my mother when she was not appreciating my successes as I wanted her too. No one had ever done this before. This is when I really started believing in Nischal. Who would take the risk to stand up to a parent if what they were saying wasn't true? In a country where I didn't know anyone, I found a deep authentic connection to someone who believed in me. As a result, the belief that I was meant to contribute in a bigger way was renewed in my heart.

My in-laws had always been progressive and open minded. They made it so easy and comfortable to adapt within the family and in India. The support was amazing and my kids learned the true meaning of a joint family. As a result, we spent ten years in India. It was incredible!

Unfortunately, at the peak of our business, my husband was travelling quite a bit which made it difficult to spend quality time together and the stress of the entrepreneurial roller coaster was so much that old and new symptoms appeared. I had to go back on some medications. During the same time in 2012, my mom was diagnosed with lung cancer. I thought that if my mom, who was so particular about health and diet, could get lung cancer, then anything could be possible with anyone. I was flying back and forth from India to the U.S. for nine months, before moving back to Maryland for the following nine months until she passed away. I was at the peak of my stress—with the uncertainty of my mother's health, the guilt of neglecting my kids and the absence of my husband. It also broke my heart to see my mother suffer. My doctor said I was a prime candidate for a heart attack or a stroke. When my mom died in May 2014, I relocated to Dublin, CA to focus on my health and the children. Over the next two years I was able to rebuild my health.

I've been in business with my husband for over 16 years helping him achieve his dream, and I never really had a connection to myself. I had become an introvert at my parents' hands, and I had followed their plan for me. Then I had been a mother and a businesswoman supporting my husband and his dream. I loved the entrepreneurial journey with my husband. I was able to support him in the way he needed, and I was shaped into a stronger, independent, sharper person thanks to Upendra's habit of throwing me into complex situations and making me fend for myself. Upendra was the blacksmith and I was the iron in the fire getting shaped. I am so thankful to him for that. But I don't think I ever knew myself. So, this is where spirituality really began to work in my life.

"Behind every successful woman is a tribe of other successful women who have her back."
— **Anonymous**

As I was exploring who I was through the journey of meeting phenomenal women in my community, I attended various seminars and meet-ups. I met a wonderful friend, Becky Diehl, who runs a forgiveness ministry with her husband Steve. Becky and Steve have been instrumental in helping me understand what forgiveness means. Although their program is bible based, I was still able to understand. Becky explained the message of God in a simple, practical manner that applied to today's life. This deepened my spiritual insights. She helped me reconnect with Hinduism and I truly began to understand the concept of God within myself. In fact, I can say through Jesus I was able to understand and connect to Hinduism better. This is a true integration of community and culture. I also began to listen to transformational leaders and coaches like Tony Robbins, Jim Rohn and The Secret team. One day when I was listening to Lisa Nichols, I learned why I needed to share my story. She said when you go through a major life challenge or solve a complex problem, the story is not yours to keep. You must share. You don't have to be a victim. You can change the meaning to be something that helps others—by telling your story.

"Always look at the solution, not the problem. Learn to focus on what will give results."
— **Anonymous**

The question in your mind right now must be what is the real solution? I believe this is going to be an ongoing exploration. Here are some suggestions to get you started. You'll need to keep in mind that everyone is unique and has specific needs. The key is to pay attention to what works for you. How well you do will depend on your commitment to practice.

- Look at holistic integrated healing. Our body is an integrated machine, and what happens in one area affects another. Holistic inquiry is to establish the root cause instead of just treating the symptoms. Sure, the medical community is crucial in our healing journey. But, we need to work as partners and be proactive rather than reactive. Functional medicine seems to address this philosophy. Find a doctor who shares your values and health philosophy. Ask lots of questions of your medical care team, and don't be afraid to get multiple opinions.

- Try an elimination diet. Start with eliminating gluten, dairy and red meat.

- Follow a clean diet. Add as many raw vegetables as you can. Eat organic as much as you can. You can even become an urban gardener, like me, and grow your vegetables on your balcony.

- Make sure your plumbing is working properly. It is important that you are expelling waste properly and regularly, both urinating and excreting. This is especially important before you detox. This happens when your gut is clean. Not passing waste is like not cleaning your fish bowl for months. Yes, it's really bad.

- Exercise consistently. What is the best form of exercise? The one you will do. The idea is to move your body. So do your favorite activity.

- Allocate sufficient time for sleep. This is when your body restores and recharges.

- Have the courage to listen to your inner compass and follow its guidance. Trust your gut and listen to your heart.

- Practice Daily Self-care and Self-love. This includes giving yourself permission to breakdown and cry

- Release emotions that no longer serve you. Open up space for new experiences to enter.

- Process unprocessed emotions. Let go and forgive.

- Ask for help. You're still a strong, respectable person, even if you ask for help.

- Stand up for yourself and make your voice be heard. This doesn't mean you have to be aggressive or put anyone else down. It does mean paying attention to your likes and dislikes.

- Reduce your stress. It's important to understand what triggers your stress and your flare-ups. When you know them, then you can actively remove them or avoid them. For a free assessment on How to Identify Your Trigger Points write to me at seema@seemagiri.com.

- Be in action!

It sounds like a lot of work doesn't it? To be honest it is, but it's so worth it! Right now you may not even believe that you can do this. It may feel overwhelming. I get it. I felt that way too. But the reality is that if you don't try, you'll never be able to do it. In fact, the very reason you should be doing this is because you don't believe in yourself enough to be convinced it will work. When you engage, you'll greatly change your confidence. The areas you resist the most are the greatest growth areas. Everyday that goes by where you don't engage in taking action towards improving your health, you're letting one more day pass you by that could have been more awesome. You might not care now, but consider this: as you lay on your deathbed and you review your life, the only things you'll regret aren't the shots you took and missed but the shots you never took that could have made your time on earth more magnificent. Not to mention that your family depends on you to make the changes that both you and they need. What legacy do you want to leave behind?

As Theodore Roosevelt says, "Do what you can from where you are with what you have!" This is actually a spiritual practice. Like Nike's slogan, "Just do it!" done consistently.

Life is not supposed to be difficult. You can get through it with ease and grace. The challenges we encounter are really there to teach us a lesson or sharpen us even more. If you stay true to your nature, life is easier and things start to fall into place effortlessly. The best analogy is that we are diamonds in the rough. The challenges are supposed to polish us so we can shine with our light; with the gift we're supposed to bring into this world. I truly believe that all of us have a unique purpose in life that is meant to be shared.

"The best way to get rid of the pain is to feel the pain. And when you feel the pain and go beyond it, you'll see there's a very intense love that is wanting to awaken itself."
— **Deepak Chopra**

Believe it or not, I consider my autoimmune disease a blessing in disguise. It forced me to reclaim my nature and voice in this lifetime, while I can still make a difference in the world. Today I'm a successful businesswoman, involved mother, supportive wife and active community member. I serve as a board member and I perform leadership roles in non-profits in my community. It gave me the opportunity to connect the dots and let me reconnect to myself in a profound way. It has also enabled me to connect more deeply and authentically with my children, husband and friends. I have thriving relationships. I'm pain free and off of 25 medications. I am down to only one and even for that, the dosage is reduced. I'm still making dietary changes. From time to time I get off my healthy track and indulge in sinful pleasures such as chocolate and ice cream. I simply get back on track without beating myself up and without judgement. I'm still learning. I'm a work in progress. Most importantly, I've found my purpose and passion. My life's work is to help women with autoimmune disease or symptoms, through …

- Personal, loving coaching to build your confidence and courage, and walk beside you through your recovery journey.

- Bridging the gap between your doctor's allopathic care and mind-body-spirit practices to create a holistic recovery plan.

- Advocating for you with your doctors and caregivers; work with your family to support you in your journey to a new life.

"The moment a woman decides to be unafraid she is transformed. When she recognizes the power and possibilities of her own strength and surrenders every fear to that power, she becomes the greatest version of herself."
— Diane Von Furstenberg

What can I do for you? As Denis Waitley says, "Time and Health are the two most precious assets that we don't recognize and appreciate until they have been depleted." The thing that bothered me the most was the time I lost being controlled by and managing my pain; time lost with family, time lost with my son and time lost where I didn't make a financial contribution to the family. While I can't recover that time, it has taught me to be more present and cherish every moment. This is my invitation to you to get your health and your time back, to design a life that brings you more control, energy, and balance. My work addresses the whole you—body-mind-spirit—and is drawn from the best practices in holistic healing, ancient eastern modalities, my own "kitchen-tested" practices and love. I want to hold your hand while you embark on your own journey of self-discovery—in the way only someone who has walked the path can. I've developed a program called "Take Charge of Your Health Blueprint for Women with Autoimmune Disease," which includes the strategies and life hacks I've created over the years. In this program you'll learn how to nourish your body and soul, how to energize yourself and how to take massive action and measure yourself based on your beliefs and standards. The point is to create simple systems that will help create a structure in your life that's specific to your needs.

My questions to you: Are you ready to break free from your pain cycle and TAKE BACK YOUR POWER? If you are ready to take charge of your recovery, then please contact me to schedule a free 30-minute Take Charge Session at seema@seemagiri.com

"There is no greater gift you can receive than to honor your calling. It's why you were born and how you become most truly alive."
— Oprah Winfrey

Thank You!

Family Is Everything

DAN ROGERS

Hundreds of years ago wooden ships brought immigrants to the shores of what would become the maritime provinces of Canada. Why did the pioneers brave starvation, malnutrition, disease or shipwreck?

Today, a number of immigrants arrived at Pearson International Airport in Toronto, Ontario. Why did they leave their countries, their jobs and friends to try and carve out a new life in Canada?

Ask such questions of either group and you would likely receive the identical answer: "To build a better life for my family," they would say. Why? Because family is everything!

In 1916 a young couple, Clarence and Lizzy, got married and boarded a train to northwest Saskatchewan. The rules were that if you were over eighteen, married and agreed to live on and work the land, the government would grant you a quarter section, which is 160 acres or 65 hectares.

At first they plowed the virgin fields with a team of oxen. The prairie grass roots were so thick that the girl had to follow along behind the plow, cutting the roots of the prairie grass with a butcher knife. Her first three babies miscarried. Then, on her fourth pregnancy, the boy rounded up just enough money for one train ticket to the closest town that had a hospital (Lloydminster). He took her in a horse drawn wagon across the prairie for many kilometers to the train station, put her on the train and returned home to continue working the fields. The girl gave birth to a healthy baby girl named Grace. That baby girl was my mother.

My grandmother was what was known as a Bernardo child. She was in a program based out of England that was founded by a man named Bernardo. Orphans and children whose parents could not afford to look after them were shipped to Canada to live on farms. Some of the families treated the child as one of their own, while others treated the child as a slave. The end result, however, was that they got to Canada. And it worked, albeit slowly. So … my mother had a better life than her mother … I am having a better life than my mother … and my son, an only child, came home from the hospital not only to his own bedroom, but to one that had a four piece en suite bathroom. Also, by the time my wife and I are gone from this world, he will be an automatic millionaire.

My hope is that you and your family can accomplish this quicker than we did. We were slow learners. It took us over a century to create wealth. But the fact that you are in Canada and reading this book already puts you in the group that is most likely to succeed. Do you find that hard to believe? Then just think of all the people who came home from work today and are either checking Facebook or watching reality TV. They definitely aren't reading a book about how to succeed financially.

THE PURPOSE OF THIS CHAPTER

The purpose of this chapter is to help educate you to use whatever money you have to benefit you and your family in the long run.

The first thing I want to do is ask you a question: What is your biggest asset? Many people will answer that question by stating what they own. Various answers will be the most obvious ones like my house, my car, my life insurance policy, my retirement fund. But the real answer is you or, to be more accurate, it's your ability to earn a living.

Now, consider that the average annual income in Canada is around fifty thousand dollars (at time of printing). That means in a typical forty year career you will have grossed two million dollars. Yet, most Canadians don't own two million dollars of mortgage free real estate or don't have two million dollars in the bank or even in an insurance policy. Why is that?

It's simple mathematics …

Mr. A and Mr. B both moved to Canada about fifty years ago from the same country. They both got jobs at the same company for the same wage. But Mr. A saved up his money for a down payment on a house and also budgeted in the monthly premium for a permanent life insurance policy, while Mr. B spent much of his disposable income on trips back to his homeland, coffee shops, take- out food, and cigarettes.

Both A and B died about twenty years ago. The daughter of Mr. A inherited a mortgage free house and a life insurance policy, while the son of Mr. B ended up with nothing. Because the child of A immediately had cash in hand, from the insurance money, and she chose to live in the house for free, she was able to invest both the life insurance money and the monthly rent she had previously been paying. Meanwhile, the son of Mr. B had to save for years and years before he could get out of the apartment he was renting, because saving up while paying rent is much more challenging. In the end, however, B descendent was able to buy a house and make some modest investments.

Eventually the heirs of both Mr. A and Mr. B died. The grandchildren of A have inherited multiple real estate properties and investment funds easily worth in excess of a million dollars, while the family of Mr. B ended up with only a few hundred thousand, as the real estate and other investments were purchased later in their parents' lives and didn't have time enough to grow. The property may not have even been mortgage free at the time of Mr. B's death.

So, the third generation of the A family are now millionaires, while the same generation of the B family has enough money for a modest down payment on a nice house.

You want to be Mr or Mrs A. Buy a home early and pay off that mortgage. Protect your ability to earn with the proper insurance policies and invest on an ongoing basis. Read on, I'll show you how to do it. But first a discussion about estate planning

WILL AND POWER OF ATTORNEY

We have been talking about estates. These are passed on to beneficiaries through the vehicle known as the will. But, over the several years that I have been in this profession, I have encountered a rather high percentage of people that do not have their wills done. And you do need one. Not a "do it yourself" will kit that can be purchased online or at a business supply retailer. Generally, the legal system does not consider this type of will to be valid. No, I strongly urge you to have a lawyer draw up your will. A good lawyer. A conscientious lawyer. Here's why …

An elderly widower sells his house, puts the money in the bank, moves to an apartment, and marries a much younger new wife. His lawyer draws up a will stating that his estate will be divided amongst his wife, his three children and his two favourite charities. The lawyer did not enquire about what type of account the money was in or ask any questions of that nature. When the man died, the executor of the estate found out that the bank had advised the man to name a beneficiary to the account, so the man, not being given a full legal explanation of the ramifications, named his wife as beneficiary. So, on his death, the bank immediately transferred 100% of the funds into the wife's name, and there was no legal recourse to get her to divide up the money according to the will. The will became a useless piece of paper. The three children and the two charities received nothing from the fund. That man was my father.

The lesson to be learned is to never assume that a professional you hire is automatically going to do things in your best interest.

Power of Attorney: There are two types of power of attorney: one for personal care, and one for property. This means that you designate a person to make decisions on your behalf should you reach the point where you can no longer make these decisions yourself. **Personal care** refers to topics such as choosing a personal support worker, a nursing home, treatments, medications, and other things of that nature. **Property** refers to topics such as whether or not to sell the house or rent it out or authorize repairs, and whether to sell the car, or cut the lawn or many other property related items.

In listing a power of attorney, remember that you do not have to have the same person for all areas. You could have a daughter who would be the best for personal care, an eldest son who would make the best executor, and a youngest son who is in real estate who would be the best person for property decisions.

I should also mention **Probate** as it is a complicated and frequently costly procedure wherein you must prove the validity of the will. The general rule is that if there is a beneficiary listed on the account, then probate is not required.

When the funds are in a bank, the money could be in one of several different types of accounts. It could be in a chequing account, a savings account, a TFSA (tax free savings account), an RRSP (registered retirement savings plan), mutual funds, segregated funds, GIC (guaranteed investment certificate), a RIF (retirement income fund), and a number of others. The bank would likely ask you to name a beneficiary on the account. This is done to prevent probate. However, remember the story about my father and learn from it. If there is only one person that you want to give your money to, then that is fine, but if there are multiple people, you must name them all.

PROTECT YOURSELF

In order to open this discussion, we need to go back to the reason everyone comes to Canada in the first place. We all know the answer to that one: to build a better life for your family. At the same time, we need to recall your greatest asset. It's you, and if you go down, everything that you worked for could be lost. So we are going to address a very important issue, income replacement. This is generally broken down into two areas; disability coverage and critical illness coverage.

Disability coverage: Disability insurance is meant to replace part of your income (usually 55%) in case of injury or illness. Now, the first thing to know is that not all disability policies are equal. Some give you the right see your own doctor—some do not. And that makes all the difference. The first group of claimants tends to be entrepreneurs who don't want to be away from their jobs any longer than the insurance company wants them to be. The second group of claimants tends to be more the corporate type, a type that encompasses malingerers—those people who are in no rush to get back to work after an injury or illness—the type that breeds distrust in the insurance companies. Make sure you're in the first group.

Integration of benefits: What this means is that if you signed up for a $2,000/month disability policy and you get hurt, and another organization also agrees to pay you let's say $1,200/month, whether it is another insurance company, Workers Safety Insurance Board, the employer, or whomever, then your insurance company only has to pay you the difference of $800/month. You can find policies that don't have this clause.

Return of Premium: What if you are lucky and never get injured? How would you like to get all your money back when you retire, tax free? Yes, there are disability policies available that have this benefit.

Soft tissue injuries/back injuries/sprains/strains: This is another very important feature. Many disability providers are so concerned about people faking injuries that they won't pay out unless something shows up on an X-ray. You don't want a policy like that. You want a policy that will cover you in all cases of injury or illness.

Injury occurs on or off the job: Many employers who provide a benefit plan to their employees will have disability coverage that only covers on the job accidents. While better than nothing, statistically, the average Canadian is more likely to get hurt in a car accident, at home, or while participating in sports and leisure than actually getting hurt on the job. That' the kind of coverage you want.

No limit on number of claims made: This one is fairly self-explanatory.

Make sure your provider does not have a clause where they can terminate your coverage if you make too many claims.

Critical Illness/Hospital Sickness Benefits: Let's imagine that you or your spouse were diagnosed with a terminal illness or a debilitating disease. The ill person might wish to do their "bucket list," go back to visit the homeland, see the Seven Wonders of the World, or take a cruise around the world. But from where would the money come? Cash in RRSPs? Sell the house? Remortgage the house? The problem with doing that is it ruins the whole game plan of coming to Canada to build a better life for your children and your children's children.

This is the reason that critical illness coverage exists in a place that already has state funded health care.

And just like disability coverage, it is possible to get critical illness coverage with a Return of Premium Clause, meaning that if you remain in good health, you get your money back at the end.

LIFE INSURANCE

There are many different types of life insurance. It is vitally important for you to know the differences so that you can pick the type that is the right one for your situation.

Reason for life insurance: Do you have massive debt from a mortgage or business loan that if all goes well you will have paid off before retirement? Or do you want to leave your family a lump sum of money for a particular purpose, regardless of whether you die young or old? These two situations require (differing) insurance products.

The standard formula that the insurance industry uses for determining the amount of coverage is: ten times annual salary plus debt. So if you make the average Canadian income of about $50,000 per year and have a three hundred thousand dollar mortgage, then the calculation would be to have $800,000 in coverage.

Term Insurance: Term insurance would be better understood by the public if it were renamed "temporary insurance." With term insurance you are buying a window of time. If you die in that window of time, the insurance company writes a cheque to your beneficiary. If you die outside that window, they cut no cheque at all.

Permanent insurance: Permanent insurance is frequently known by its official name, whole life insurance. If the reason for buying is that you need some security to pay off your debts if you die young, then term is the way to go, but if you want to leave a lump sum to your family whether you die next year or in sixty years, then you will want a permanent product.

Term to 100: Term to 100 is a rather unique type of life insurance that is sort of a hybrid between term insurance and permanent insurance. As we have already read, the disadvantage of a term policy is that it eventually runs out, but the advantage is lower premiums. The disadvantage of whole life coverage is that the premiums are high, but the advantage is that it lasts forever. What if you could get a policy that never runs out but that has the lower premiums more associated with term insurance? Great, right? That's why many companies don't offer the product. But you can find it, if that is what you want.

No Medical Insurance: No medical insurance is frequently called other names such as final expense insurance, funeral insurance, burial insurance, guaranteed issue insurance, instant issue insurance, and perhaps a few other names. It is frequently advertised by way of television commercials, and mail flyers delivered by the post office. The target client is often a retiree whose term insurance has now expired but who still wants to leave a lump sum when he or she dies. People with health problems who will never qualify for standard application coverage also tend to buy this type of policy.

Universal Life: This is another type of whole life policy. It can be a bit complicated, so I'm going to give a brief explanation of this product here. With a universal life policy, a portion of your premium goes into an investment. Over the years, the idea is for the investment to grow substantially. A universal life policy with a face amount of $100,000 would have an additional investment portion attached to it, so after a few decades the policy might pay out in total $150,000, $200,000 or more. Although this seems like a great idea, low interest rates over the past several years have made many people who hold a universal life policy realize that the projected payout at the end is going to be considerably lower than what the agent had suggested way back when the policy was first taken out.

The moral of this story is to make sure you sit down with a financial professional who will do a "needs analysis."

PLANNING FOR RETIREMENT

RRSP stands for Registered Retirement Savings Plan. An RRSP isn't an investment, it's a shell in which you can store all sorts of different kinds of financial plans and investments.

An RRSP could contain stocks, bonds, mutual funds, segregated funds, Guaranteed Investment Certificates, syndicate mortgages, Guaranteed Investment Accounts, just to name some of the more popular products that a typical Canadian RRSP might contain.

What an RRSP does is let you defer income tax. It is designed for Canadians who know that they are going to be bringing in less money after they retire than they are currently bringing in now. Canada Revenue Agency (CRA) charges income tax on a sliding scale depending on the income of the person. Someone who doesn't earn much income may pay no income tax at all, where someone with a high income might pay out 40% of their pay to income tax.

Life Income Fund: A life income fund generally comes from a company pension. Some employers offer a company matched retirement plan, meaning that whatever you put into it, they will contribute an equal amount. When you leave the company, it is recommended that you do something with it. The reason is that if the company runs into financial trouble, your retirement fund could be gone, or at least reduced. It has happened before, and will most likely happen again. Instead, if you quit, get downsized, or retire, you should move that money out of there and put it with an investment firm. That way, the success of your former employer will have no influence on the fund.

Various investments

Mutual funds are what are known as securities. The agent or broker must hold a license regulated by each provinces securities commission. Mutual funds are really just a collection of various stocks. They were designed for the purpose of the small investor being able to get into the stock market without a large cash outlay and with a lower risk. There are thousands of different funds out there, and virtually all of them are quite heavily diversified. This is both good news and bad news. The good news is that if one or a few of the companies that are inside that particular mutual fund take a huge nose dive, it won't cause your fund to drop too dramatically. The bad news is really the opposite side of the same coin. If a few of the stocks in the fund soar tremendously, your fund won't go up all that much because of all the other stocks in there that remain steadfast or have dropped. Mutual funds have no guarantees whatsoever, so if your fund dropped way down, you have only two choices: you can cash out at a loss, or you can hold onto it for enough years and hope that it rebounds satisfactorily. Mutual funds are also subject to fees known as Management Expense Ratios, or MER. If your fund's MER is 2%, then on a one hundred thousand dollar investment, expect to pay two thousand dollars per year in fees.

Segregated funds are very similar in concept to mutual funds. Segregated funds are sold by life insurance companies. Many financial experts describe segregated funds as "mutual funds with an insurance policy wrapper". Segregated funds must be kept separate from the insurance company's regular finances, hence the name. A "seg" fund and a mutual fund may both be investing in the same stocks, the main difference between the two, is there is a guarantee with a seg fund. The guarantee in a seg fund is generally either 75% or 100% of the original investment, depending on which plan you take. That means that you are guaranteed to get back either 75% or 100% of your money, even if the fund loses money. You will have to hold onto the fund for an agreed upon length of time, usually ten years to get this guarantee. And it is important to know that this guarantee is not free. A seg fund will have extra fees associated with it to cover this guarantee. If you cash out before the agreed upon time, you get what is in the fund, whether it has gained money or lost money, less any fees. If the seg fund rises in value, most plans will allow you to "reset" the guaranteed amount to this higher amount, however, that would mean that doing this will reset the amount of time, usually ten years, that you must hold the fund.

Depending on which plan you take, 75% or 100%, if you die while the funds are down, your beneficiary will receive 75% or 100% of the fund.

Guaranteed Investment Certificate (GIC): A GIC is a savings account where the interest rate is pre-set. There is an amount of time, generally two years, three years, four years, or five years that you must keep the money in the account in order to obtain that interest rate. If you withdraw the funds earlier than that date, you won't get the agreed upon interest rate. The longer you keep the money locked up, the higher the interest rate you can get.

Guaranteed Investment Account (GIA): The simplest way to describe a GIA is that it is like a GIC, except it is carried by insurance companies, just like seg funds, and the guarantee activates in the event of the contract holder's death.

If the contract holder dies while having a GIA, the company guarantees the highest of the two following things: either the balance of the account on the date of death; or 100% of the sum invested in this account.

Syndicated Mortgages: A developer who wants to build a condo tower, a commercial office building, or any other large construction project can generally only get conventional bank financing up to a certain percentage of the cost of the project. The remainder of the amount he needs has to come from someplace else. When you agree to give the developer your money, you go on title, the same way that your bank is on title for your house, if you have a mortgage. Syndicated mortgages have been around for a long time, but ordinary folk like you and me have only started hearing about them in the past few years. The reason is that they used to be reserved for those with very large sums to invest, like a million dollars. It was only relatively recently that the industry opened up the market dramatically by lowering the minimum investment to twenty five thousand dollars. Generally, the syndicate mortgages that have come across my desk pay 8% per annum, simple interest. It is important to know the difference between simple interest and compound interest. With compound interest, you receive interest on your interest, but with simple interest you do not. A typical syndicate mortgage locks your money away for a period of time, frequently three or four years.

Gold and other precious metals: The only reason that I am even mentioning this topic is because I am told that there are people on the radio urging us to buy gold. On the financial security pyramid or pillars, or ladder, or however you would like to refer to it, precious metals are to be considered at the top, right up there with collecting works of art. This means that it is something that would be recommended to do after your house is mortgage free, and you have amassed considerable wealth and assets.

REAL ESTATE

Buy vs Rent: There are always those who debate whether or not it is better to rent and invest more in the market, or buy real estate, and subsequently have less money left over at the end of the month to invest. Remember that home ownership has two entirely separate goals. The first one is to make money on it, either by buying low and selling high, or by making improvements to the property, thus increasing its value, or by paying off the mortgage so that you no longer have the expense of making payments. The second goal is to improve your quality of life. You have your very own residence without being at the mercy of a landlord, should they decide to sell the property, or raise the rent, or move into it themselves, or move a relative into it. You also have total control over what colour you would like the walls painted, the types of light fixtures, window coverings, faucets, countertops, and a host of other features.

Buying Real Estate: The first thing you will require is the **minimum down payment**. When you buy with less than twenty percent down, this is what the banks refer to as a high ratio mortgage. This requires you to have mortgage default insurance. The most popular organization the banks use to obtain mortgage default insurance is the Canada Mortgage and Housing Corporation (CMHC), a crown corporation. Two other companies that offer this are Genworth Financial Canada, and Canada Guaranty. They will charge a fee, and blend it into your payment. This can only be avoided by having a minimum of twenty percent of the purchase price of the property already saved up and available. For a first time home buyer, this could be difficult. Most of the property purchases I have made had CMHC on them. I still found this to be the lesser of the evils when compared to paying rent.

Next, you will need to **obtain approval for the mortgage**. You should do this before looking at any properties. There are two ways of doing this. The first is to talk to your own bank branch. The second is to use a mortgage broker. The advantage of using a mortgage broker is twofold. First, they do all the work, don't charge you and get paid a referral fee from the financial institution where the mortgage is placed. The second advantage is that they will frequently work with multiple lenders, giving them and you more choices. One thing they will be looking for is your Total Debt Service Ratio (TDSR). This means that all your payments, mortgage, utilities, and other things such as car loan payments and line of credit payments should not exceed approximately forty percent of your overall gross household income. So first of all, you should not be considering real estate if you owe any money on anything else, and yes, that includes your car.

The next thing is your need to have established a **credit rating**. There are two credit rating services. The most popular one is Equifax, and the other one is TransUnion. You can obtain your credit score from these institutions yourself at no charge. They will probably try to get you to pay for it, and they will quite likely offer you the information instantly if you pay, but you can wait and get it the slow way without having to pay. If you are new to the country, or young, or both, you may not have established a credit rating. The first thing is to have a credit card. Obviously, the intended goal is to pay the balance off every statement, thus avoiding any interest payments. If you think you can get by in this world without a credit card, you thought wrong. Not only is it vital in establishing a credit rating, but without one, it is generally quite difficult to purchase anything online, obtain tickets for a major event, rent a car, book a flight, stay in a hotel, and a host of various other situations that will cross your path from time to time.

Types of properties: There are really only four: condo, townhouse, semi, and detached

Condo is short for condominium. You will usually see them in the form of high rise buildings, but there are townhouse condos and even detached condos. With a condo you only own the inside, the condo corporation owns the outside. I'm using simple terminology here. You pay a monthly fee to them and they are responsible for exterior things like the roof, landscaping, snow removal, elevators, and really everything this is not inside your unit.

The next type of property on the scale is the **townhouse**. They can be condos or freehold. If it is a townhouse condo, you pay a fee to the condo corporation, just like a high rise, and they look after the same things like the roof, snow removal, and grass cutting. If it is a freehold, you own the whole thing, and you are responsible for everything. The main items to think about with a townhouse is that you share your walls with someone else.

Next on the list is the **semi-detached**. This has all the same possible downsides as a townhouse, but you are only sharing one wall. The key to a good semi is to have a great neighbour on the other side of the wall. But of course, you have very little way of finding that out until you are already moved in.

A **detached house**, meaning that it is not connected to any other building (you can walk all the way around all four sides), is the ultimate goal, in my humble opinion. In many regions, especially in the Greater Toronto Area (GTA), the detached house is sought after not only for the buffer zone between neighbours, but because many of these houses are ideally suited to having a separate basement apartment with a separate entrance, frequently a side door. This is an excellent way to bring in extra money to offset the high mortgage payment.

GOVERNMENT RETIREMENT BENEFITS

There are five main areas about which you will need to know: Canada Pension Plan (CPP), Canada Pension Plan Survivor Benefit, Canada Pension Plan Death Benefit, Old Age Security (OAS) and Guaranteed Income Supplement (GIS).

The Canada Pension Plan (CPP) is something that you would have paid into during the course of your working career. You can apply for it as early as age sixty or as late as age seventy. If you apply for it at age sixty, you will, however, receive a 36% reduction in benefits. If you apply for it at age seventy, you will get an increase of 42%.

According to the government of Canada statistics as of the year 2015, the average CPP monthly benefit is $619 and the maximum is $1,065.

Old Age Security: The Old Age Security (OAS) is a benefit for which you can apply at age sixty five, as of now, however, there are plans to increase the age at which you can apply to age sixty seven. Time will tell if the federal government sticks to the plan of age sixty seven, or if successive governments decide to roll it back to age sixty five. At time of publishing, the OAS is around $565 per month, however, it is indexed to inflation, so it generally goes up a few dollars per month every year.

CPP Survivor Benefit: If you are the first to die in a spousal or common-law relationship, the surviving spouse should apply for this benefit. It is generally 60% of the deceased partner's monthly CPP benefit, or if death occurs before age sixty five, then this benefit is calculated on the amount that it would have been if death had occurred at age sixty five.

CPP Death Benefit: Only a very few countries offer this benefit. To be eligible for your estate to receive this benefit you must have made contributions to CPP in the lesser of: one third of the calendar years in your CPP contributory period, but no less than three calendar years; or ten calendar years.

The amount of the death benefit depends on how much and for how long the deceased contributed to the CPP. The maximum benefit is $2,500. According to the latest statistics, the average benefit is around $2,300. The CPP death benefit is calculated as the amount equal to six months' worth of your monthly CPP benefit.

Guaranteed Income Supplement (GIS): If you live in Canada and have a low income, this monthly non-taxable benefit can be added to your Old Age Security (OAS) pension, if your annual income (or in case of a couple, your combined income) is less than the maximum annual income. The Canadian government calculates this maximum annual income amount based on numerous different criteria such as if you are single, widowed, or divorced, or if you have a spouse that receives the full OAS pension, or if your spouse does not receive the OAS, or if your spouse is already receiving the GIS and the OAS. You can always go the government's website yourself when you need this information: www.servicecanada.gc.ca

FINAL ARRANGEMENTS

This section will be dealing with an area that most people are not particularly thrilled about discussing. Furthermore, most people are not willing to walk into a funeral home and ask questions. Fortunately, I worked in the industry for ten years, so I'm in the position to not only help you spare your family a lot of grief and hardship, but at the same time, save you money as well.

There are two ways to pre-arrange your funeral: One way is to pre-arrange but not pre-pay. The other, and more preferred way, is to pre-arrange and pre-pay.

Cremation verses Burial: The main reason that 90 % of the people I have talked to about funerals over the years choose cremation, is so they can avoid the cemetery completely.

If you choose cremation, there are five options open to you regarding the disposition of the remains.

1. Your family can take the urn home with them and put it on the shelf. (This is not for everyone, some like the idea, some hate it.)

2. You can have the ashes scattered. Note: this choice is completely legal.

3. If you have an immediate family member that is already in a cemetery plot, most cemetery boards will allow you to place your urn in your family member's plot, generally for a fee of a few hundred dollars.

4. You can purchase your very own plot and have your urn buried there.

5. Cemeteries have structures called columbariums, or wall niches, that you can purchase for the purpose of having your urn placed there permanently.

Funeral Service Choices: For the sake of simplicity, there are really only three.

1. **A Direct Disposition.** All this means is that you are hiring the services of a licensed funeral director to send a transfer vehicle to your place of death, whether that is a hospital, a nursing home, or your own home. They will pick up the remains and transport them back to the preparation room at the funeral home, arrange for the cremation and return the ashes to you.

2. **A Memorial Service** contains everything a direct disposition contains, but the funeral establishment puts on a service, either in their own building, or in the church of your choice. Sometimes people want it to be held in a different location, such as a club that has their own facilities. It is important to note that with a memorial service, the body is not present, no casket is present, cremation has already taken place, and most often, the urn is present in lieu of a casket.

3. **A Traditional Service**: This is the type of arrangement where the casket is present. I'm not sure why, but many people are under the misconception that a traditional service is not available with cremation. The facts are that there are only two real differences between a traditional service with cremation to follow, and a traditional service with burial to follow. The first difference is that with burial, there is a funeral procession from the funeral home or church to the cemetery, and with cremation to follow, there is not, because the body has to be transported to the crematorium. The second difference is that with burial, a casket

is purchased, and the casket is buried. But with cremation, the funeral home usually provides the use of the casket for the visitation and service, and hidden inside the casket underneath the white satin lining, where no one can see, is the combustible, rigid, leak-proof container that is always necessary with cremation.

"I'm donating my body to science!"

This is what you need to know with regards to whole body donation. Medical schools, or schools of anatomy will accept body donations to train future medical professionals. It is completely different than donating organs. The body must be in very good condition and there must be a need for the body. It is important to remember that if you have a pre-paid funeral and you are accepted by a medical school, the pre-paid funeral fund will be returned to the family with interest.

SUMMARY

What do all of these things I've been talking about have in common? The greatest point of all that I've written here is that there are many ways for you to achieve wealth and grow it. An early mortgage and long-term investments can result in a free home for your loved ones to live in, money for them to live on and funds to grow even more money. They can even take the money they used to pay rent with and purchase yet more investments, so that when the third generation matures, there is a literal fortune waiting for them to inherit.

We also discussed investment vehicles such as real estate, mutual funds and term deposits, touching on various types of each, the idea being to make you aware of the choices you have moving forward. We even talked about how to protect your earning potential with disability insurance and life insurance. The chapter ended with a looked at funeral planning.

You came to Canada to make a better life for your family. This chapter can set you on the proper path to achieve what you wish. Good luck in all you do!

Save My Relationship

The Master Plan for Creating an Amazing Relationship

CHRIS HART

Beata came to me with her relationship in tatters. Her boyfriend, Matt, had recently moved out of the flat they'd shared for five years, claiming that he no longer loved her. She thought they had been moving towards marriage and was utterly devastated, lost, and confused. She told me that I was her last option. I hear that a lot. Beata did not believe that she could rekindle the relationship with Matt. She thought it was a lost cause and that she was a lost cause, too. She was grasping at straws. I saw a woman whose self-esteem and confidence were at an all-time low. I saw a woman who was broken, emotionally. I saw a woman I could help.

I welcomed Beata with open arms. We sat down and, as I listened to her talk, I formulated an action plan for her to follow. She stuck with the plan, and with me, through many months of emotional healing and relationship work. I am thrilled to say that Beata and Matt are now happily married! Beata succeeded because she realized that she needed to work on healing herself as well as her relationship. Do not think this was an easy task for Beata. Some of the things I had to say were not easy for her to hear. My job is to be real. I will not tell you what you want to hear; I am not here to stroke your ego. Healing does not occur within denial. Beata had to do some difficult self-healing before we tackled her relational-healing with Matt. She is now extremely confident and aligned with her feelings. Furthermore, she is happily married and pursuing a life of "happily ever after."

If you are struggling with a failed, or near-failing, relationship, I can help you, too. My methods are not traditional self-help methodology, which focus on the mind. My methods focus on the heart; I concentrate on emotional guidance. You did not enter into your relationship using your mind. On the day you met your mate you did not think to yourself, "He seems like a good fit. I think I'll develop a loving relationship with this one." No, you did not use your mind; you used your heart. You met and fell in love. Therefore, you cannot solve relational problems with your head. This is an emotional problem that requires heart healing.

Maybe you wish to rekindle a romance that is dwindling, but you aren't quite ready for marriage. Such was the case with Talia, who came to me during a troubling time in her life. She was young and in love...or so she thought. Her boyfriend, Doug, had recently distanced himself from her. At first, he pulled away emotionally. He still hung out with her and took her out, but he seemed distracted and was not fully present with her. Eventually, he began making plans that did not include Talia. She was left feeling hurt and confused. Talia's thoughts began to take over her conscious moments with a constant barrage of questions: Was Doug the right choice for her? Should she wait for him to come around and decide what he wants and who he wants to be with? Should she move on and date someone else? Exactly what was he doing when he was not with her?

Talia's friends were divided. Some counseled her to not let Doug get away; they gave her ideas of how she could change herself to be more attractive to Doug. Others scoffed at that notion and told Talia she could do better than Doug, and counted off several other guys who'd already expressed interest in dating Talia. Talia's mother told her that "Things have a way of working themselves out" and to be patient. Talia's head was spinning from overthinking this situation.

Talia eventually got out of her own head and contacted me. After our first session, Talia was able to organize her thoughts and set them aside to focus on her heart. Soon she realized that she was not quite ready to give up on Doug. She was not sure if the relationship was one that would last forever, but she wanted to pursue it. So, we set to work.

I soon realized that Talia was harboring quite a bit of anger, not only towards Doug, but towards the friends who had been so quick to tell her what to do. Of course, this really means that Talia was angry with herself for allowing others to treat her this way. She denied this in the beginning; I had to be quite stern with her to enable her to see how she was allowing others to treat her. Talia was young, a college student, so her friends held a lot of influence over her. So often I find that people care more about what others think of them than what they think of themselves! Eventually, Talia came to see that she had to stop listening to others and only listen to me, and herself.

We put an action plan in place and Talia was able to examine her heart, rather than being lost in her thoughts all the time. After working with me, Talia was able to emotionally heal herself. She is now a much stronger young woman who has many close friends, yet thinks for herself. Thanks to my work, Doug has decided that he wants to continue his relationship with Talia. He is much more open with her about what he is wants. Talia and Doug are now happily dating and are excited to see where their relationship goes in the future.

When you utilize my methods you will find the last missing jigsaw piece that solves everything in your world of romance; that is, your relationship. I will enable you to regain your confidence and self-esteem by giving you the knowledge of what you can do to resolve your romantic problems. Many women come to me for help. My methods work because I am a man, therefore I think like a man. I can help women understand how their men think.

One of the first things a woman does when her relationship hits the rocks is to pick up the phone and call her closest friend or family member. After all, your friends will commiserate with you and offer you a shoulder to cry on. On the other hand, be cautious because your loved ones may soon begin to belittle your man or point out everything that was wrong with the relationship. This is no good! Whether they are correct or not, they are not in your shoes. They are not living your life, nor do they understand what you feel or what you want. You should stop listening to friends and family, especially if what they are saying does not align with your desires. They usually mean well, but cannot understand your relationship or your heart.

Once you stop listening to others, you must next stop overthinking. Putting an end to overthinking is the key! If you are hurting and mourning the loss of your love, you are thinking, thinking, thinking about what you can do to get him back, or what you wish you had done differently. You are spending too much time and energy thinking about your problems. All of this overthinking is surely affecting other areas of your life. Are you able to be productive at work? Or do make careless mistakes along the way because you are focused on your current loss. Are you fully present when someone else is talking to you? Or is your mind on your own problems that you are feverishly thinking about? Are you losing sleep due to overthinking? Overthinking about your current romantic problems leads to self-blame, loss of confidence, and a lack of awareness of the true nature of the problem. Two people usually share the blame when a relationship ends. When you overthink, you victimize yourself. Do not think like a victim. I will teach you how to become a victor. With my new way of thinking, you will be put back in control of your emotions.

Having control over your emotions is the key to victory. I will teach you how to have closure with the old self and to be the woman in control. Controlling your emotions can change you completely. You may not recognize this change in yourself, but others will see this metamorphosis and be inspired by you. People will be attracted to you because of your inner transformation. Learning to become the victor and think like a victor requires that you get real with yourself. You must look deeply into your own desires and motives to recognize things that need to be changed. Consider me your personal coach; I will "kick butt" if I sense that you are being too soft on yourself, just as any good coach does with his or her trainee. I want you to succeed, therefore I will not accept anything less than 100% from you. If you are just looking for someone who will stroke your ego and tell you that you are always right, you may wish to go back to your friends. I am not that person. I am the person who will affect real change in your life and in your relationships.

There is beautiful change to be had, if you are willing to make it. If my relationship were ending, I would be wondering what I could have done to change things or save the relationship. Regrets would always be there somewhere. Women with regrets cry. Do you have regrets? Successful women do not cry; they try. In fact, they make things happen. Women who take action have no regrets. You, too, can make things happen to solve your relationship problems.

When a woman comes to my practice, the first thing I ask her is this: Do you really want him back? This may sound like an empty question, but it is not. The answer to this question is incredibly important. Often, women do not know the true answer to this question when they first come to see me. If you only want him back in order to exact revenge on him for the way he treated you, my methods will not work. You must be sure that you want him back and that you want him back for the right reasons. The second question I ask is this: To what degree do you want this man back in your life?

Sometimes a woman comes to me and does not know the answer to those questions. I met with Carla and could tell right away that she was unsure about seeing me. She was unsure about many things. Once we cleared the air with incense and began to set aside her thoughts and focus on her heart, Carla realized that she held too much anger and resentment towards her boyfriend to continue a relationship with him. She had been blinding herself to this reality because she was afraid of what to do without him.

Carla was so afraid of being on her own that she was willing to chase after a failing relationship. She was so caught up in her thoughts that she did not even realize what this was doing to her heart. Carla was putting herself last and discounting her own feelings!

I quickly formulated an action plan for Carla. She chose not to pursue the failing relationship with her boyfriend; rather, she chose to pursue the failing relationship with herself. I got real with her and coached her on how to put herself first in her heart. This does not mean that she was to become a narcissist! No, this meant that she had to re-learn how to love and care for herself. She also had to learn to let go of her boyfriend. Using my methods, Carla was able to heal herself emotionally.

Carla recently contacted me to let me know that she is dating someone new. She is in love! She breathlessly told me how her new beau was the perfect match for her. I smiled to myself because I know he is the perfect match for her because she healed herself and was open to finding love.

Maybe you will decide that you do not want your man back in your life. Maybe you will decide that you want your man back for the right reasons and you realize to what degree you want him in your life. I can help you with both situations. When you work with me, I ask that you listen only to two people: yourself and me. Please do not think I am being conceited with this statement. If you are having a problem with a guy, listen to me. I do not say this to sound conceited, but I am a guy. Since I am a guy, I think like a guy. You need someone who thinks like a guy to help you with your guy. Furthermore, I have your best interest in mind. I have no preconceived notions about your relationship or whether the man is 'good enough' for you. I want what you want.

Listen to yourself. Have you been doing that? Or have you been overthinking the problem and assigning all kinds of blame to yourself? Listen to your authentic self. Do not allow others to influence your thoughts. It matters what you think and what you want, not what the others in your life think or want. Once you are ready to stop overthinking and blaming, you are ready for productive change.

I will share a bit of what I can do with you to save your relationship. First, I use incense to clear any negativity in the air. I know which incense to use that will combine the right energy with the right purpose of healing your relationship. Incense also prepares your mind for the process of healing your relationship. The incense I use will heighten your awareness, focus your thoughts, and bring about calm or healing energies during our work. When using incense to enhance energy, it provides assistance to direct your energy in a specific direction of self-healing. You will ultimately be able to alter your inner perceptions about yourself to create the life you want. Of course incense cannot do this alone, but it can help create or enhance the desired energies for our work together.

Along with incense, I use crystals in my practice. Crystals have the power to heal and attract if used wisely. Rose Quartz is a particularly good crystal for healing relationships, and is one that I use in my practice. Rose Quartz, also known as the Love Stone, is the stone of unconditional love; therefore, it is particularly powerful for healing broken relationships. Rose Quartz opens the heart chakra to encourage forgiveness and will, along with my counseling, help you let go of anger, resentment, jealousy, or any negative feelings you have towards your partner.

We begin with the first of two tests. These 'tests' will determine my unique action plan for your situation. The first test involves the use of imagery. Imagine your guy standing right in front of you. Take time to allow his image to materialize in your mind, noting details of his appearance. After you have the image of him in mind, ask yourself what colour you feel he has near his head area. Next, ask yourself what colour he has in his heart area. Finally, ask yourself what colour he has in his erogenous area. Take your time and allow the colours to materialize. Now take a look at yourself. What colours do you see in these areas for yourself? If you are struggling with this imagery while reading, do not lose heart. When you visit with me, I will guide you to accurately see the colours you have in mind for yourself and your partner.

Colour is, at its most essential, light and energy. People have been using colour, along with light and energy, to heal for thousands of years. Colour is also a form of nonverbal communication that influences emotion. There is a specific psychological response to each colour. Psychological effects have been observed relating to the following two main categories of colour: warm and cool. Warm colours, such as red, yellow, and orange, can spark a variety of emotions ranging from comfort and warmth to hostility and anger. Cool colours, such as green, blue and purple, often spark feelings of calmness and peace, as well as sadness or melancholy.

The colours you saw in the above exercise indicate your emotions regarding yourself and your mate. Your colour choices guide me in developing your personal action plan to harmonize the colours into the proper colour for a successful, loving relationship. If your colour choices indicate that your relationship is in real danger of ending, I can work with you to change the colours you see.

I will teach you to use your mind and emotions to align your proper colour with your guy. Along with incense and crystals, I utilize a picture of the person, since a photograph is an inner vibration of a person. Once you start working on your colours with me, relational changes occur quickly. A woman I counseled recently was able to complete an emotional bonding with her guy, even though he had moved out and ended the relationship. This couple is now married.

I hope that I have inspired you to take action to salvage a hurting relationship. If you are ready to take charge of your life and save your relationship, contact me through my website: www.loveguidance.co.uk. My hope is that reading this has been an awakening for you to see your own problems as they truly are, and to stop thinking like a victim. Through a session with me, you will be able to regain your strength and confidence to win him over. I will help you find closure with your old self and what has gone wrong in your past. Your new way of thinking will attract people to you and put you back in control of yourself and your emotions.

Do not be a woman with regret; be a woman in control.

Gender Balance & Win

How Leaders Overcome the REAL Obstacles

SUE JEFFERSON

THE CHALLENGE FOR MEN AND WOMEN IN BUSINESS TODAY

Today's world of business has come a long way though it is still lagging behind in gender bias.

As a woman how do you navigate this issue and ensure success in your workplace, become an exceptional leader and love both your work and your home life?

As a leader, male or female, how do you enable your organisation to become naturally inclusive, overcoming the unconscious bias that commonly exists?

Many successful companies have adopted programs to recognize talented women, create an inclusive culture and are designed to nurture their success driven employees. This is a wise move for companies looking to make an impact as these high achieving individuals can have an enormous positive effect on business results.

The reasons why diversity & gender balance brings better business performance are obvious – they bring breadth of thinking to every leadership team. However, biases and barriers can still exist even in the most innovative and progressive companies, particularly if they are quite male orientated. These barriers manifest either as unconscious bias; emotional reasons that are not recognised as such, or with a limited few, still conscious bias that are now simply hidden under the auspices of legislation, but don't let that be an excuse for what's holding you back.

This chapter, compiled from listening to and reading the very many different viewpoints of business leaders, head hunters, men and women, as well as my own experiences as a Boardroom executive who has delivered unprecedented growth, seeks to offer those leaders of companies with an unconscious bias together with their HR Directors, a way to recognise barriers in their organisation, practical solutions to overcome them and how to get started in creating and benefiting their business with gender balance in their workplace.

A PRACTICAL SOLUTION FOR LEADERS AND INDIVIDUALS

Using my 30 years work experience, where I became one of the first female

Director/VPs in a global food manufacturer, leading multi-discipline teams and transforming business outcomes, all while maintaining a marriage of 24 years and raising a family, I have created a toolkit called the C.A.R.B.O.N. Way to Transform to Sparkling Success ©. I now work with visionary organisations to enable their high potential women to develop simple to apply strategies & support leaders to constructively address these barriers and provide practical applications to enable mutual success and career/life balance.

First of all, what is this toolkit that I talk about? Known as the C.A.R.B.O.N. Way to Transform to Sparkling Success© with six key pieces, addressing the most common barriers holding back women and organisations.

Cutting Through To Be Heard: If you are not heard by your colleagues and superiors in the workplace it will be difficult to achieve any level of success. Before you do anything you must first be heard.

Influencing Action - Getting the right actions from the right people: Once you have caught the right ear you need them not to just listen but also put your words into action. Without action you cannot move forward and accomplish goals.

Resilience - Responding to Setbacks: You are going to face them and the higher you go, the more you'll have, and the more significant they will be. Setbacks happen to everyone but it's how you respond to them that matter and pave the road to success in both work and life.

Resilience - Building your Mental Toughness: Underlying resilience is an important asset in today's competitive business world. As moving up in the workplace and standing out in the crowd becomes harder, mental toughness will give you the ability and advantage to stay strong, balanced and be an inspiring leader.

Creating Awesome Self Belief: This is something that I find alongside Cutting Through to Be Heard and Influencing Others, that women struggle with the most. Being skilled in this, is the backbone to enjoying work everyday, being bold to make a difference in your organisation and having the ability to develop others.

Setting Outcomes and Wowing People - As you deliver unprecedented results and inspire others to deliver too: Most people do not think ahead to outcomes but just focus on the tasks to be done. It is much more powerful if you start with the end in mind, determine what is missing to achieve this and then plan the right deliverables. It's faster, more likely to secure success and engages people to deliver for you. At a mastery level this will enable you to transform everything you touch.

Our Needs: Knowing the human needs that drive behaviour and how to use them. This is important because these unconscious needs underpin everything you do and everything that other people do. Understanding these, means you can enable your own and others' needs to be satisfied, feel fulfilled and so sparkle inside and out.

So that's the C.A.R.B.O.N. model©.

For maximum impact and embedding new ways of working, I bring the model to life as an in-house workshop for organisations who want to develop their high performing, high potential talent. If you keep these concepts in mind through the rest of the chapter where we discuss the barriers women face, the unconscious barriers holding back leaders and how to address them, I have no doubt in my mind that you will find the mutual success you are seeking. I look forward to every woman in an organisation using these concepts and becoming a sparkling diamond very soon.

UNLOCKING PROVEN BUSINESS BENEFITS FROM GENDER BALANCE

Technology is changing the world and how we view it, quicker than ever before, from employment to leisure and transportation to education. With such rapid change, as customers change the dynamics of business rules and organisations struggle to maintain growth, why are more leaders not tapping into a proven source of greater performance?

A source that McKinsey & co. stated is worth an additional $12 trillion of business, in their May 2016 report "Women Matter: The business and economic case for gender diversity" Technological moves over the next 15 to 20 years will bring a wave of changes that will fundamentally change our careers. This $12 trillion opportunity comes on the back of gender balance within the world of work, where gender gaps in our society are closely tied with improvement of access to areas that could unlock economic opportunities for women.

However, barriers do exist. It has been said, the danger of the modern gender workplace bias is that too often it can seem like no problem at all. The disappearance of explicit sexism can give the false impression that it no longer exists. Studies spanning over the last few decades indicate gender bias not only exists but thrives in male dominated professions. A woman meant to be a leader, will stand her ground where she pushes through this narrow minded viewpoint that they are second class citizens and sometimes wins, proving her worth. Astounding research results reports this stereotype gender bias is thriving and the experiential evidence is additionally overwhelming. Many actions have been uncovered that women can take to position themselves for the career advancements they have worked for and deserve. Although stressful for a woman in the workplace they need to be aware of the negative gender stereotypes found in most job markets surrounding them. When they make their career decisions they need to anticipate the biases some of these stereotypes foster; and they need to manage the impressions they make to avoid or overcome these biases. Women, as well as men need to know what their desired outcome is and pursue it in whichever manner necessary to achieve their goals.

Performance and business success research has taken the focus and attention into the female entrepreneurship field although there is still much controversy on how to measure performance. This is over which indicators should be taken into account, but mainly when there are comparative studies between men and women entrepreneurs. This ludicrous controversy in today's world seems even more difficult to imagine as it is sexist but exists. At its essence, it is about the success of a company. Posing the quandary of whether a company can be successful if they are created by women, or have a higher rate of failure or lower performance in comparison with those created by men.

Economic performance studies have used variable ways to measure it between the women and men, without considering other type of measurements that can be important for women entrepreneurs, apart from the economic ones. However, when researched using more than the economic results of performance it has been argued that male and female entrepreneurs pursue different business goals. Entrepreneurial women generally emphasize social goals, while male entrepreneurs emphasize economic goals.

Research studies conducted tell us that companies with at least one woman on the board outperform those companies that had no women. They indicate blue-chip companies with at least one woman on the board outperform others with no women by 26%. The study was done over a six-year measurement by Credit Suisse (Credit Suisse Group is a Swiss multinational financial services.) Studies also show results that the difference made by women during the financial crisis was particularly noticeable. New growth was strong in mid-decade as there was little difference in share-price performance between companies but by 2008 after the financial crisis (2007-2008) stocks with women on the board have strongly surged ahead. It is reported by securities research and analytics that greater gender diversity is a valuable additional metric to the financials, when evaluating investments.

Another astounding indicator, where studies over a six year period reported an average return on equity of 16% with companies that had women on the board vs. 12% from those that had none. These same companies with women reported the income grew 14% on average over companies with no women on the board at 10%.

Further investigation into outstanding business performances and gender bias find that there is a large opportunity cost for companies associated with male-only executive boards. Like a world still addicted to fossil fuels, these companies are suffering now. The conclusion drawn is that those businesses stuck in the past are not fully unlocking their growth potential.

In today's fast changing environment, large companies need to find ways to become agile, understanding and responding to the dynamic needs of their customers and delivering the best solutions ahead of far reaching competitors. Frankly, without gender balance and diversity, those organisations will become case study dinosaurs.

It is clear from this evidence that gender balance makes smart business sense.

Business management teams at all levels need to change from limited Group Think to broader thinking and can do so by better leveraging their hidden advantage with their female employees. Some obvious benefits from gender balance include smarter understanding of fifty percent of purchasers (the females): their issues, their needs, their drivers for response. Intuitive understanding of employees and their needs enables better communication, engagement and support for ongoing change. Broader diverse experience enables people to see challenges differently – identifying different risks and creating different solutions.

The final advantage is that by working in a collaborative way and delegating outcomes not simply tasks, results can be achieved at a better pace.

A significant benefit of gender balance is that these improvements often come from employees already within their system. There will be hidden talent within everyone's current organisation – women who know the business, systems, the people, the vision, how the company works. Some of these women will be evident in the talent review picture as high performing and high potential people. So once unlocked, given the right opportunity and support, they will hit the ground running and your organisation will see improved performance within months.

Additionally, the natural behaviour that arises from gender balance is improved collaboration – seeking to find win-win situations, building on others' ideas and putting the company success ahead of their own. Including female employees in decision making, replacing dated Command and Control management methods, is a necessary requirement for an organisation to leverage the maximum of benefits from their employees. Not only will gender balance and collaboration improve morale across every level of management team, the cultural change will start to subdue some of the behaviours seen between ambitious executives which leads to the fragility of the boardroom which is a challenge for most CEOs to manage.

As organisations see improved prosperity, risks better managed, stronger morale and commitment, they benefit from a natural cultural shift which will create better team working and an agility to act in a way that every large organisation desires if they are to successfully respond in this fast changing world. A more accommodating workplace, enabling work and life integration and balance, is becoming a must for the new generation, male and female, therefore a company that embraces this now will not only benefit from the immediate advantages but will be advantageously placed to secure the best talent going forward. Equally they will embrace diversity and be a natural global player, attracting customers across cultures.

BARRIERS FOR LEADERS BEYOND THE RATIONAL

Why is it that despite these clear and known benefits to gender balance that many organizations are still hesitant to implement these changes?

These barriers arise from several common but unspoken fears from leaders. Feedback tells me no-one is calling these out. Without recognising these are real concerns and sharing how visionary leaders are boldly tackling these, progress of organisations and individuals will not be made.

Here are the 6 most common fears of current leaders:

Meetings: "My leadership team is difficult enough to manage, with different egos, ambitions, inability to share concerns in case of perceived weakness… adding in an unknown quantity of a female will create chaos/ risk loss of control (and I cannot tackle these in my usual man to man way or places)"

Emotions: "I do not know how or want to deal with a person who cannot take criticism, face tough challenge, respond to setbacks or have issues outside work being brought into work."

What ifs: "Managing the hassle for projects, for clients, for replacement and handovers when a female takes maternity leave, and additionally the unknown void if she is to return. Accommodating part time or flexible working arrangements and the additional responsibilities means her mind will no longer be 100% on the job."

Flexibility: "It is critical that tasks are completed on time and to the highest standard. Also it is essential that clients can always reach the person they require and teams can access individuals to progress actions and decisions at pace. This is a major risk if I must offer a female flexible working arrangements and even more in circumstances when a person needs to unexpectedly look after a sick child or relative."

"In accommodating flexible working, I risk ending up with so many people working different part time hours that it becomes incredibly difficult to manage holiday cover and workflow for the organisation."

Am I a bad person: "If I raise the issue of diversity and our need to improve, this implies we are not equitable now – I will therefore be labelled as sexist and I, my department and company will be perceived negatively."

Possible Traits: "I value those I work with, but knowing the demands at the highest level, I believe women do not have the stamina for long hours when a project deadline is required, the mental toughness in a crisis or ongoing hard knocks. They will not be taken seriously by colleagues due to lack of ferocity or presence, lacking commitment to make unpopular decisions. They juggle too many balls and cannot focus or as an opposite cannot control the degree of ferocity and directness which is uncomfortable for colleagues."

How does an individual or company overcome those barriers?

The following sections address these concerns directly:

ACTIONS BY VISIONARY LEADERS

Meetings: Not many CEOs voice their common struggle in leading a team of highly competent but all male, ambitious people who think alike but play political games to advance their own success and agendas, fearing openness as a sign of weakness that will be exploited by others. Feedback suggests these boards are far more fragile than one would assume from the outside, indeed some are even dysfunctional. Highly effective teams are those with high degree of trust and collaboration, who share commitments to advance the organisation first, are willing to share their concerns, make requests, meet promises, build with ideas to support a colleague's success, are aligned to decisions made in the boardroom and consistent in conversations inside and outside with all people. Successful leaders set out their expectations of their team, both collectively and individually, raising the bar, understanding concerns, positively and consistently enforcing it when new behaviours (or old behaviours) come forward in the meeting room.

Great leaders today are not expected to have all the answers but instead be good at asking insightful and probing questions whilst seeking suggestions from others. The introduction of any new member of the Board (male or female, internal or external appointment) causes change as positions are assessed and reset, so this is a great opportunity for leaders to refresh everyone as to their vision, expectations, ways of working, share purposes both for the organization and individuals, then structure agendas and separate conversations to enable dialogue to cover all elements that move situations forward (People, Possibilities, Plans, Performance & Produced actions)

Emotions: CEOs should allow themselves the luxury of continuous development. So many Boards struggle especially when asking for change by the rest of the organisation, when the employees will tell you, it is the management team that are the dinosaurs. A culture of ongoing personal and team development including the top is something that differentiates the Great from the average. Great CEOs encourage this ongoing learning – both individually and collectively.

Understanding and influencing people is one of the skills that creates unprecedented success and is never complete. Understanding people and what makes them fly, what makes them struggle, how they inter-relate, how to lead them, when knowing that there are so many different types of people, is invaluable.

Women fall into a range of types too. The women who have shown themselves to be high performers are the ones leaders want to have playing key roles in the company if they wish the organization to be sustainable.

Using the people techniques available through the many great training companies, it is very rewarding to have the skills to unlock what makes people tick, manage previous avoided conversations in a non-confrontational way and to see people transform and develop the areas they need to strengthen. I'd recommend www.paracomm.com, www.h2h.uk.com, as well as myself at www.realisepossibilities.com and www.boardroomreadywomen.com

Let me be clear – there are plenty of very talented women who possess all the demanded skills to lead and create unprecedented success, engaging colleagues and workforce as they do it. It is a talented CEO who can uncover and sponsor such women.

What ifs: Career planning, life planning are good conversations to have with line managers ongoing at quarterly reviews. When this is done, few surprises arise and company and employees can plan and accommodate changes in a mutual way for things such as succession planning and handovers. Equally, contact days when on maternity leave are beneficial. Like with flexibility, two way solutions can be found when planning a return. Returnies to work are often better than new recruits – as they already know the company, the systems and the people.

Flexibility: Flexibility is fast becoming a demand of the next generation, male and female, whose attitude to work and life balance is very different to the standard mindset we are familiar with. Therefore approaching this in a way that brings advantage to your company, attracting the best talent whilst ensuring the business needs are fully met, is a lever visionary leaders are keen to embed.

The basis is to have Flexibility as a two-way thing – enabling the company and individual needs to both be met. Seek mutual solutions to achieve business outcomes (the what) as opposed to being limited by traditional ways of working (the how). Have a method where the individuals suggest specific flexible working ways to meet their needs whilst making sure that company concerns and needed solutions are found together with a shared commitment to making it win win. There are lots of suggestions in HR guidelines that shape mutually reasonable conversations. This department is also useful to maintain an overview of all the flexible working so the collective solutions also stay workable.

Evidence shows that when flexibility is offered, alongside mutually agreed conditions, the organization and leader gain 120% of that individual's loyalty to deliver and excel for them, especially when it matters. Better still, it creates a culture where all individuals feel valued and this builds to the strongest team commitment and outputs.

Am I a bad person: Voicing what you stand for, as a future vision, is evidence of a strong leader, a driver of positive change. It is important to state that any current situation is not WRONG or Bad but what's MISSING is an opportunity to leverage how better gender balance can bring the organisation improved results.

Be ahead of the curve as at the time of writing, new UK/EU legislation is requiring organisations with more than 250 employees to publish their pay & bonus gaps between gender. This public information will prompt fresh assessments of company image and their leaders. As a global issue, the pressure from customers, clients, shareholders and future talent will build and build.

Possible Traits: Irrespective of gender, people must demonstrate they are leaders first, although beware reinforcing the dated traits of Command and Control as the organization will not be resilient to change and will become a dinosaur whatever the gender balance. Women may naturally show some skills which the organization needs, whilst not show some of these additionally desired traits. All this can be quickly and easily trained. Upon being made aware and experimenting with them in a development workshop, leaders will know if they can leverage them like many other skills.

Remember the objective of gender balance is that a blend of skills from men and women are brought to each leadership and management team, to create better thinking and better decisions.

It's an Individual leader's journey first, followed by the organisation's journey to success that leads to the culture changes required for gender balance. This culture shift involves moving from group think to broad think, going from the invisibility of talent to talent fully leveraged, limiting attitudes and behaviour to enabling attitudes and behaviour and going from circular conversations to transformation conversations.

These barriers begin as conscious bias – "I don't value women in the workplace", "I am not going to accommodate and I shall make decisions that discourage" (eg. starting a meeting at 6am to "prove" business is no place for the working mother!).

As the culture matures they shift to unconscious bias – all the barriers and probably more, that I listed as common but unspoken fears (evidenced by women retention at the middle to higher levels being low).

With a leadership mindset to change and actions applied, as I've highlighted here, the culture changes to conscious inclusion and with enough consistent reinforcement, you will naturally move on to world class, unconscious inclusion.

This will stand you head and shoulders above your competitors, your employees will be your ambassadors and together with stronger, agile performance you will attract your chosen clients, shareholder investors and have the pick of future talent. All building a sustainable future.

THE WATCH OUTS

It is important to also know what not to do.

These are based on my observations but not all people are in agreement.

Do not have **quotas**.

Always fill positions based on merit; Quotas have unintended consequences including undermining existing talent in leadership roles.

I see several companies set a % target but NOT time bound. The organisation does everything it can to balance the genders at all levels. KPIs measure progress to balance.

Actions include, advertising posts where females will most likely access them not just the usual trade journal. When vacancies arise, CVs may be assessed blind. The recruiting manager must write to the Board indicating if and why they've chosen a male candidate over a female one. There is visibility as to each department's gender balance, at all levels and pay gap differences. No-one wants to be bottom of the league table. It equally ensures the balance is not out of kilter the other way around – too many females is not good business either.

Do not avoid **conversations about gender.**

Making assumptions about what high potential women do and don't want without discussing with them, is foolhardy; Having honest conversations to explore future plans and find flexible solutions so no compromise in delivery of critical outcomes or client support is ideal. These should be with all employees, all genders and life stage. You can read the details on planning for these conversations in my book Boardroom Ready Women.

Raising the topic with an incumbent Board and creating the vision for change maybe where you need to start.

Do not **dismiss comments.**

Purporting to listen but dismissing concerns over colleague comments or behaviours, head in sand rather than dealing with grievances, leads to poor corporate culture and an undercurrent of mistrust and no loyalty. Beware of having a written policy that is not enforced. I see far too many Diversity and Inclusion statements in company's annual reports or on their websites alongside the overused phrase "people are our most important asset". However the % gender profile rarely matches the polished words.

Walk it, don't just talk it.

It is always powerful to ensure that concerns both from men and women are acted on and used as opportunities to reinforce the desired culture.

Do not leave Gender Balance to be the **responsibility only of the HR department.**

This is everyone's responsibility and a leader's accountability. Of-course use the skills and resources of this specialist function to co-ordinate the many elements required to create this culture change but delegating the outcome to one department and a Chief HR Officer, is doomed to fail.

STEPPING FORWARD

How can your desired cultural shift get started?

It is best to engage a few trusted advocates to steer the process.

Make stated the intent to leverage the advantage of gender balance.

Ask the right questions to establish where you are and collectively shape where you want to be (not quotas but targets without a time limit).

Then identify high performers and high potentials from talent reviews.

Initiate a programme of tailor made development support for these identified females and to educate and engage your mixed gender leadership teams. Combine this with your mainstream people insight support from HR. Highly recommended of-course is my proven successful workshop programme from www.RealisePossibilities. com or www.BoardroomReadyWomen.com.

In parallel, review or create policies and procedures and engage all leadership groups.

Seek out and recognise effective behaviours and outcomes that drive change especially in performance reviews, succession planning and recruitment.

Finally secure ongoing feedback from the women, the men and the leaders about what to Keep doing, Start doing, Do differently and Stop doing.

The final thing I should say, is whilst there are a lot of unconscious biases and barriers that boardrooms might have today, particularly if they are quite male orientated, don't let the culture change of an organisation have to be complete before seeing the appointment or promotion of a high potential woman. In my experience and feedback from the workshops I've run, 80% of the solution lies within action that can be taken by an individual.

Women can even be holding themselves back, but with this practical and effective C.A.R.B.O.N. Model toolkit, immediate awareness and change can be seen, benefiting the individual woman and the business area they work in, immediately. They can start overcoming their immediate barriers. Really, there is nothing stopping anyone.

If we encourage all leaders to understand the root cause of challenges in diversity and inclusion, introduce the application of practical solutions that enables them to establish gender balance in their workplace, they will see the benefits and fast.

All businesses, governments and people are talking about this but are hitting barriers and not succeeding in overcoming them. This is because they offer rational solutions to unconscious emotional barriers. I am trying to change the dialogue. My motivation is driven by a desire for better business performance, improved economic success and to see a balance with women also reaching positions of greater influence thereby creating more opportunities to improve their social environment & encourage the next generation.

Simple smart business sense.

Every individual woman who becomes familiar with the C.A.R.B.O.N. Way to Transform to Sparkling Success © will recognise the barriers they face in the corporate world and now have a practical way to address these barriers, enabling them to move forward and be a catalyst for their success and their organisation.

Not everyone wants to be or is capable of being a leader and that's OK. For those that do (especially women), we need encouragement and techniques to unlock their natural talent and also overcome barriers they face. I do not believe there needs to be a choice to sacrifice home life or career, as you can love and succeed with both if you create clarity, efficiency, priorities, self belief, belief in others and have great tools to assist you.

I believe, and have seen it and done it myself, that there are actions that you can take at every level in an organisation, to become a better leader, and become boardroom ready. Boardroom ready does not mean every woman should be or will be a Director or a Partner in a business, or that they even want to be, but embracing these practices will also enable individuals **to perform better** in their current role. It will create more enjoyment in the workplace, more fun and balance with loved ones, and generally an **ability to live life to the full.**

Whether you are that woman, that visionary leader or HR catalyst, you can make a difference in this, one of the most important of business topics today.

Above and Beyond

DR. MARYLYN POYNTER

"Retirement at sixty-five is ridiculous.
When I was sixty-five I still had pimples."

- George Burns

When I hit retirement, I honestly thought that life would be amazing. I had spent many years as a dental surgeon and now I was looking forward to enjoying life, my way.

At first, my retirement fund seemed fine but a few years in I realised that my pension was not allowing me to live the life I dreamed. I had wanted to do things with my husband, but I also had kids and grandkids that I

159

wanted to do things for and support.

I felt frustrated and trapped. What was I going to do? Go back to work? I had already spent a lifetime working. This was supposed to be the time for me to do what I wanted. The other option was to continue as I was, always juggling my wants and needs. Not being able to live my dream and leave money for the future generations.

Neither one appealed to me.

Do you feel that way? Like you have no choice but to accept the way your retirement is going and hope that there may be something left over when you pass?

What if there were other options? What if you had a choice? What if you could set goals and reach them? That is what we are going to explore in this chapter. Many retirees I have talked to are living lives of quiet desperation when they don't have to.

I decided to do something about my situation and researched my options. Can I admit something to you? It was pretty daunting. What could a woman of my age do? Going back to school to learn a new trade was not feasible, plus, who would want to?

I could get a part-time retail job but to me that seemed like moving backwards after all my years of being an educated professional. Plus, I valued my free time, and there was a golf course with my name on it.

What else could I do? Then an idea came to me. I googled it and my first thought was, "Maybe." I always try to keep an open mind and be courageous enough to try new things.

Want to know what it was? I was considering running an online business. Are you shocked? I was, and I was the one considering it.

Have you considered working online and then came up with all the reasons why you can't?

Do any of these reasons sound familiar to you......

1. Too Old to Learn the Technology

Aren't computers, websites, and online shopping for young people? There is no way you can learn those things They are way beyond your skills. You will look so foolish. People will laugh at you and think you are stupid for even wanting to try.

2. Isn't it Expensive

By the time you get everything set up, isn't it going to cost a lot of money? How do you know that you will get that money back? You have some money, but you can't afford to lose it. How long will it be before you are making money? These are all questions people ask themselves.

3. What to Choose

If you google, "How to make money online?" the options are endless. How do you choose? Which ones are scams and which ones are shiny objects that distract you from your true course. All these questions need to be answered.

But for me, learning how to do things online was different. I have always been one who sees the goalpost, moves towards it and just as I reach it, move it back. I want my life to be one of forward motion where I am always learning and growing. So, I chose to do something most people my age wouldn't even consider; I started learning how to set up a business online.

Was it easy? No. Did I require help? Yes. Did I make mistakes and get caught up in shiny object syndrome? Yes. Yes. Yes. I spent money on trainings and programs that were a distraction, but almost two years later I am making five figures, travelling, enjoying time with my family, and partaking regularly in my favourite hobby, golf. Life is good.

How was I able to do that? I put aside my doubts and my pride and I learned how. I tried new things, asked for help, and spent a lot of time on YouTube (what an amazing website, you can learn anything you want on there for free,). I outsourced some things and, most importantly, I got the professional coaching, training, and support that I needed to succeed.

MY CHALLENGE TO YOU

You have a choice. You can continue to live the rest of your life struggling financially, not being able to live a full, fun life. You can watch each day go by wishing and hoping that things were different, looking at your kids and grandkids knowing that there is nothing that you can do to help them.

Or…

You can take my challenge and become an online entrepreneur. Now is the time to silent those voices in your head that are giving you all the reasons why you can't succeed. We grew up in a generation where we were taught to be average, to do what everyone else was doing and not to expect anything more.

We were conditioned not to take risks because they might backfire, and people might think we are strange. We can't have that, now can we?

"The biggest risk is not taking any risk... In a world that is changing really quickly, the only strategy that is guaranteed to fail is not taking risks."
— Mark Zuckerberg

It is time for something new. What if I could show you a way to earn money online? Would you want to learn more? Of course, you would. Here's the thing. If I can do it, so can you. I didn't start this process with great computer skills. I could do the basics but beyond that it was all a mystery to me.

When it comes to learning how to run an online business you have three options:

1. Figure it All Out Yourself

This is how I started. It is the hardest way to go. I spent hours upon hours in the beginning just trying to figure out what business I wanted to do. Then I tried to learn the basics, but it was hard. Easy terms that young people know and understand were like a foreign language to me.

Google and YouTube became my new best friends, but it was such a long process to do the simplest things. There were times I was so frustrated and wanted to quit. Thankfully, I didn't.

I also invested in a lot of training programs that promised the moon and the stars but never delivered. I was excited each time because I was sure that this one would work. I invested time in studying it only to realize that it was just another shiny object, all brilliance and no substance.

So, can you learn by yourself, yes you can. However, although there were many things I learned to do myself, the process was long and tedious, and during that time I wasn't making any money. Which leads to option two.

2. Paying Someone Else to Do It

There are three problems with this solution. First of all, to do everything you need, it is costly. If you don't have a lot of disposable income at hand you will either get very low-quality work or you will have to save between each step.

Second, trying to find honest freelancers who produce quality work and truly care about your project is hard. Sometimes, you go through and pay two to three people before you find a good freelancer and that is wasted money. Third, if you don't know what you are doing, every time you need to make a change you will have to pay someone to do it.

So, if you have the money, this is an option for you (provided you have the time and patience to build a good team of people to help you).

3. Work with a Professional Coach and a System

In my opinion, this is your best option as it incorporates the other two. A professional coach will be able to identify your strengths and weaknesses quickly and guide you to the best resources available to build the business that you want.

A professional coach knows all the ins and outs of running a business online and can help you both avoid the pitfalls and take advantage of the secret loopholes to success.

Their goal is to help you reach YOUR goals and YOUR dreams. What could be better than that? Someone who is on your side and can show you the ropes, will be there when you get discouraged (because you will), and help you navigate the big, wide, online world.

I am going to share a secret with you. I have found a professional coaching system that is economical (under $100USD), gives you a simple 21 step program that is easy to implement, and, on top of that, assigns you your own personal coach who is there to help you each step of the way. (http://marylynsblog.com/something-new.)

I also have some other resources that can help you in your journey to creating an online business. Check out this free PDF I created to help you with your first steps: http://marylynsblog.com/perfect-retirement

Plus, I also have my blog, marylynsblog.com, where you can find lots of free training.

I encourage you to take charge of yourself. Create the business that gives you the freedom to live the life you want and to be a blessing to your family.

I am so glad that I chose to try and didn't give up until I figured it out and now I want to help others do the same.

In closing, remember what Walt Disney said, *"All our dreams can come true, if you have the courage to pursue them."*

For FREE training go to www.marylynsblog.com

How to Gain Abundant Wealth

KAY EVE

This advice is aimed at two groups of people – first, those who heard the name of God but have not taken further action and second, those from a practising Christian background who have lapsed.

If, however, you are an atheist then the teachings described here cannot help you. I wish it were otherwise, but I cannot change how the universe is. Without belief, you cannot have God's spiritual help in your search for wealth and wellbeing. Without belief, you must rely on only human knowledge to see you through the difficult times.

The issue is that Christian teachings are haunted by two very wrong ideas. Firstly, the notion that suffering is good for you and that we must each "bear our own cross". One such example is that Mother Theresa of Calcutta refused medicine to patients in her "hospitals" because of the belief that suffering was "good for the soul." This was not the Middle Ages, but only 20 years ago, showing how deeply embedded the idea that "suffering is good, yet pleasure is dangerous" still is within Christianity even to this day. I won't deal with this idea here extensively other than to say that there are many churches that will tell you the good news, that God wants us to be happy – and what's wrong with being happy? I advise you to visit an evangelical church. The worst that can happen is you'll have a good laugh.

The second wrong impression within Christianity is that it is wrong to long for material gains. Jesus famously overturned money changers' tables in the Temple. He said "it is easier for a camel to go through the eye of a needle than for someone who is rich to enter the kingdom of God". I hope to show that what God hates isn't making money, but acquiring it dishonestly or hoarding it all to yourself. Instead, Christian teaching encourages us to live a comfortable life with your loved ones and to do good with the excess. This interpretation is often ridiculed as "praying for money", particularly by spiritual people who I want to reach. Good people also deserve to succeed! So I ask you to keep an open mind, and to give me benefit of a doubt and give careful consideration to what I have to say.

I'm certainly not saying that the Bible tells you that if you ask for gifts from God then they will just fall into your lap! Many of the good things that Gods gives us are quite unasked for – sometimes things will just come miraculously. However, what the teachings say is that if you ask, He will help you to help yourself. You will have to supply the hard work for financial success or personal happiness, but God will be right by your side.

Read on and discover God's love for us all. I know in my heart that if we start looking closely, we can find messages of encouragement that God gives mankind, messages that have mostly been covered over or shunned. I'm here to try and bring out the truth, that God wants us to know His desire for everyone to be happy and have a meaningful, fulfilling life.

And so, I thank God every day for everything that was created directly by Him and indirectly by humans in our world. I am so grateful to be here amongst all of you today.

THE GREAT DISCOVERY

When we think of our galaxy, we know that it is shaped just like a fried egg with the yellow yolk in the middle and a disc of white surrounding it. In the outer edge of the disc is our sun, with one of its planets that we call Earth, which is found to be a safe place for all living things.

During the 19th and 20th centuries, scientists gradually discovered how the universe and the earth formed and evolved. The human race had already been running around planet earth for thousands of years, living and breeding on the planet quite successfully when at peace but killing each other in times of war. Those ancient people had no knowledge of how the earth was formed, but still some of them knew the wealth teachings, and so they came to be wealthy and successful.

If you look at the world's religions today, the only faiths that teach us how to live with Abundant Wealth are the teaching of the Torah for Jews and the Old and New Testaments for Christians. The Abundant Wealth teachings were recorded in all the books we call the Bible, within which one can acquire the keys to unlock wealth and happiness.

More and more people are now searching for words of guidance from the sages of old and from modern businessmen and businesswomen alike. One may not realise that the roots of the valuable teaching from modern day "coaches" actually originate from Christian doctrine. Most people in our modern world do not know how to use and apply the keys successfully to their own lives. But through keeping in mind these teachings and keys, it is possible to achieve your goals and attain wealth, success, happiness and wellbeing.

The only thing that can maintain an abundance of wealth, success and prosperity is God. He has played the biggest part in all our lives whether we realise it or not. People can say they don't believe in God, but if they do, they won't have access to His teachings for success. A lot of people believe in other religions, but abundance only comes down to us from the most powerful, the most almighty, the most gracious and the most merciful one called God. The truth is that there is only one key in the universe and God himself has the key. By praising and asking God for His Abundant Wealth's codes you will learn how to apply the codes for yourself and become successful in every aspect of your life.

The simple question is how to become wealthy? If you believe in God, you will discover these Abundant Wealth's codes and be able to use these codes to unlock for yourself whatever your heart desires, in your personal life, business, work or family. When you have learned this, you will have learned the secret of one of the most satisfying experiences of life. You may say "Well, that's okay for those who already know God, but what about people that do not know or have never heard of God before?"

If you happen to be later, that is ok; it is very easy to join this group of enlightened. By way of illustration, I will call it a club. As you already know, if you aren't a member of a certain club, you cannot receive the access, knowledge or privileges which members can. To be in God's presence is like being in God's club just like the other Christian or religious sects' clubs.

With God we have free will to choose to worship Him or not. That is your personal choice. God does not need anything from you except to receive your sincere love and your worship. God does not want you to sacrifice anything to Him. He has already sacrificed his own beloved son Jesus Christ for us over two thousand years ago.

Firstly, you need to believe that there is such a thing as the Supreme Being who is commonly referred to as "God", with His own special holy names by which He would prefer to be called. Without this belief, you will not have your wealth key's codes to work. If you do not believe that God exists, then why in the universe or on earth would you expect any of His Abundant Wealth's codes to work for you?

Secondly, endeavour to believe that God has the power to grant you your Wealth codes to unlock the doors of the universe and give you all aspects of success and abundant wealth. God can indeed be reached directly, for there is no distance between Him and His Son.

If you are not in God's club you are an outsider, you will not receive full wisdom to understand all of God's instructions laid out before your eyes. As Jesus has told his disciples in Mark's Gospel,

Mark 4:12 Jesus said, *"When they see what I do, they will learn nothing. When they hear what I say, they will not understand. Otherwise, they will turn to me and be forgiven."*

The "forgiven" word here means to be freed from wrong decisions, wrong choices, etc. So your faith in Jesus will make these mysterious passages, the codes, clear.

EVERYTHING IS POSSIBLE

First you need to do everything physically and mentally possible to make a good connection with God!

When we discover that we are known and understood by God, it can be a very profound and moving experience. Sometimes your spouse or best friend may know or understand you on the surface, but deep down you may feel like you are alone. And yet no matter how well you are known or understood by others, no one can understand you better than God himself. As King David has put it;

Psalm 139:1-4 NIV
"O Lord, you have searched me and you know me. You know when I sit and when I rise; you perceive my thoughts from afar. You discern my going out and my lying down; you are familiar with all my ways. Before a word is on my tongue; you know it completely. O Lord."

If you believe that God exists in the world like the ancient people of past times did, then you will want to worship the Almighty for the successes in your life. But how can you actually get a real and intimate connection to Him? The sincerity of your heart is the key to success.

Three steps to Calmness:

1. Find solitude with God, away from other people and distractions. By shutting out the sights and sounds around, you will make it easy to tune in with God.

2. Find a comfortable position, select a chair or a corner of your bed. Go to the same place at the same time in the same position every day. Consistency is of the utmost importance.

3. Before you begin, relax and take a few deep breaths. Let your mind be quiet and your body relaxed. When your mind quietens, you may know

the conscious presence of God that says "Be still and know that I am God." Psalm 46:10

Now you are ready to start making a connection.

Three Steps to Listening:

1. The first step of prayer is to praise God, such as by citing the Lord's Prayer as in Matthew 6: 9-13. Let your prayer begin by praising God and you will soon find yourself in a frame of mind with Him.

2. Let some positive thinking and praying enter your mind. The secret of success is thinking and believing positively, and the same is true in prayer.

3. Ask Him to speak to you and tell Him about the things that matter to you. Whatever problems or difficulties you have, you can rely on Him for comfort, stability and the material things that the world has to offer. Once you have things off your chest, remain quite still and relaxed and listen!

By modern standards in the developed world, very few of us are really suffering. The atheists down the street will probably have all they need and live physically as well as you, perhaps even a little better. Yet, if you ask God, you will receive more blessings than they ever will and be in a better place with a better quality of life, with all the things you ask for that can be truly beneficial to you.

EXPECTING THE UNEXPECTED

Secondly you must believe that he has the power to help us and wants to help us all!

When you have asked God for the things I have described above, one final step remains - the "receiving in advance", or the assurance that your prayer will be answered. You need to thank Him and to strongly assert your confidence that He is going to provide the answer to your request. Filling your heart with positive thoughts will help to ensure that God will allow these things to happen.

Yet, how can you be assured that a constant relationship with God will produce answered prayer? The answer lies within the Abundant Wealth codes, within the heart of answered prayer, and within the following everyday Bible verses, such as;

Matthew 17:20
If you have faith as a grain of mustard seed, you shall say unto this mountain, "Remove from here" and it will move. Nothing will be impossible for you." (The "mountain" in this parable of Jesus means one of our life's great crises.)

Matthew 21:22
If you believe, you will receive whatever you ask for in prayer.

Mark 21:24
Therefore, I tell you whatever you ask for in prayer, believe that you have received it and it will be yours.

However, do not mix up the word "Faith" with "Belief". To believe that God can answer and is able to deliver all of the things being asked for in prayer, this is not faith. Everyone can have faith. The prayer of faith means trusting in God to do something but truly believing in God means to know that God is honest and will do what He says He will. It is to believe unhesitatingly that He is on the verge of doing it and that even now, the answer is on the way to you.

Many people also misconceive faith as desire, but this is false. Many people want success, but longing, wanting and desiring success is not faith. Desire, rightly directed, can produce faith and may lead you to faith, but in itself it is not faith. When you have known God intimately, you may experience a genuine re-dedication of your heart, only to be disappointed that your prayer went unanswered. This is because God may judge that the "good" thing was not what you really need at that time. He will give you something else that's good, something that benefits your life.

Faith is a common commodity. Everyone has faith. Atheists have faith that there is no God. Animals and pets have faith in their masters. Children have faith in their parents and we have faith in our Governments to watch over our nation. It is only faith in God through truly believing in Him that will reward you with your heart's desire. As James says in James 1:6-8;.

"But when you ask God, you must believe and not doubt, because he who doubts (unbelief) is like a wave of the sea, blown and tossed by the wind. That man should not think he will receive anything from the Lord, he is a double-minded man, unstable in all he does."

Believing is an act of total trust in God; it doesn't require information, knowledge or certainty – only the free and joyful surrender in His goodness. To help with this, look for the "invisible" gifts of God. They are clearly seen in the many good things that have already happened, things that are usually taken for granted. However, God alone will not change the course of some worldly events. For instance, He doesn't interfere with situations in which people have created chaos around themselves. They must deal with the consequences of their own actions. God is very constant, but for victims caught in the chaos He will turn things around for those who have the absolute trust in Him.

Each code of Abundant Wealth is laid out in the Bible for anyone to read. It has rarely been used before because few pay attention or even try to find out the meaning that God has given freely to everyone. Established religions tell people that praying for money or success is the sin of "avarice", yet churches get rich while their congregations are told to be content with what they have. But who can build a hospital or invent a new medicine without money? It is not the money that is inherently bad; it is the people that do bad things with or for it.

Most modern day sages who have written books about God's wealth codes have hidden the source of these gifts, saying that they come from the universe instead of from God Himself. One can ask for wealth, success, love and happiness until your tongue hangs out, but you will not receive the answer without asking only God himself.

Asking others who pretend to be God for favours will end in disastrous results for you, even if it may appear to be beneficial at first. Many rich and famous people have made deals with others but there is a steep price that must be paid for this false hope. Through Jesus Christ, we have paid already and there is nothing to fear when asking for success, as long as it is done without wickedness or dishonesty.

If you are still skeptical about the wealth key's code then it will not work for you. I wish you good health and happiness, but if you remain doubtful you might as well throw this book away! To have everything that you need and desire you must make a total surrender of your heart, your love and your belief to God, the powerful and the almighty who has created this world and the universe. As is said in Hebrews 11:1-6;

"Now faith is being sure of what we hope for and certain of what we do not see .... By faith we understand that the universe was formed at God's command, so that what is seen was not made out of what was visible .... And without faith it is

impossible to please God, because anyone who comes to him must believe that he exists and that he rewards (Abundant Wealth to) those who earnestly seek him."

THE TRUTH REVEALED

Who is "God" and what's wrong with the idea of a general "Supreme Being"?

God defines Himself as the great lover of mankind, and many Bible verses reveal the depth of this love.

Jeremiah 9:24
"I am the Lord, I show unfailing love, I do justice and right upon the earth; for on this I have set my heart"

Jeremiah 31:3
"I have loved you with an everlasting love; I have drawn you with loving kindness."

Mark 11:29-33
"A new command I give you: Love one another. As I have loved you, so you must love one another."

Most religious texts, Hebrew and Muslim alike, give many names of God in their own Language - seventy-two in Hebrew and up to ninety-nine for Muslims. The only one that God told Moses directly is found in Exodus 33:19. "I will call out my name, Yahweh" ("The Lord"). Even so, there are many other names given to God which reflect the compassion, kindness and generosity He had for different peoples, such as;

Yahweh-Jireh Lord will provide

Yahweh-Rohi Lord is my shepherd

Yahweh-El Shadia   Lord Almighty

Yahweh-Shalom	Lord of peace
Yahweh-Rapha	Lord of healing
Yahweh-El-Olam	Lord everlasting
Yahweh-M'kaddesh	Lord who sanctifies

As mentioned in the Old Testament, no one can see God face-to-face and live to tell, due to his vast and glorious power being too much for our bodies of mere flesh and bone. For this reason, when God appeared to Moses He covered Moses' body with the shadow of His hand.

Exodus 33:19

"I will make all my goodness pass by before you. For I will show mercy to anyone I choose, and I will show compassion to anyone I choose."

Exodus 33:20

"but you may not look directly at my face, for no one may see me and live."

As we know from the Bible, God created the universe, the world and all living things on it. Among these creations was the Sun, which produced the light and heat that God commanded to shine upon the Earth as God had wanted from the beginning.

Genesis 1:1 & 31

"In the beginning God created the heavens and earth...And God said "let there be light."

And so, humans were born on Earth in multitudes, and from them God selected the nation of Israel and the Jewish people to work with Him. Much of the Old Testament tells of God's love towards this nation. Yet men were disobedient and uncaring towards God, turning away to worship frightful and false gods instead. And so the New Testament tells us that God sent his son, Jesus Christ, to be born as a human among us and so that we would love and worship him again. As the Bible says, if we accept that Jesus is our Lord and the son of God, then we become God's adopted children and have the right to call him Father and to ask for his Wealth Keys.

Matthew 7:11

Jesus says, "Ask and it will be given to you; seek and you will find; knock and the door will be opened to you.....which of you, if your children ask for bread, will give them a stone.....if you, then, though you are evil, know how to give good gifts to your children, how much more will your Father in heaven give good gifts to those who ask Him."

So what do we know about God so far? We know we can ask Him for help in all matter of things and that nothing is too big or small for Him to handle. We can ask Him for guidance in all of our problems because He truly cares, and we can also ask him for whatever we desire and it shall be done for us. If we know God intimately and are not happy with our present situation, then we can always ask Him to change it for the better. We must remember that there is no god other than Yahweh-God who proved his love for us by laying down his own son's life for our benefit. The people who get their prayers answered are just simple people like you and I. We must never doubt in Him and we must always rest assured; God is real. He was, He is and He will be in everyone's life.

THE ASKING

But how can you actually go about asking God for Abundant Wealth?

Everything is possible with God for those who love Him. You can trust in

God that all that you ask will be fulfilled before you draw your last breath on earth, no matter how long it takes. An example can be seen in Luke Ch. 2 where Simon, the old Jewish prophet who was full of devotion to God, asked that he might meet the Messiah in his own lifetime. God answered his wishes and promised Simon would meet him before he died.

Luke 2:27-29

Led by the spirit, Simon went into the Temple. So when Mary and Joseph came to present the baby Jesus to The Lord as the law required. Simon took the baby Jesus into his arms and praised God, saying "Master, now you are dismissing your servant in peace according to your promise."

It is God's will that his children will possess Abundant Wealth and all that they desire. And so we now need to concentrate on how to build a relationship with God in order to receive his true blessings. Like any relationship, one has to dedicate oneself to make it happen. Though it is common knowledge that true human relationships are not always easy to maintain, it is different with God for he loved you first. He longed for you to love Him back, and it is up to you now to do your part.

There are only a minority of people who have a true belief in God's love and will see a miracle happen to them in their lives. It is hard for most people to love and believe in God, especially being surrounded by modern technology where things must be seen, heard, touched, felt or sensed in order to be real. God and belief in Him have become almost a myth, but the key to finding true belief is to discern God's love in your own life, which can be done in Five Steps.

1. Ask God to step into your heart and reveal his truth to you. You can do this anywhere or any time as long as it feel right to you. Once you have accepted God and Jesus into your heart, you will become an adopted child of God and you can begin building the relationship.

Revelation 3:20

Jesus says; "Look! I stand at the door and knock. If you hear my voice and open the door, I will come in, and we will share a meal together as friends."

2. Begin worshiping and praising God, whether out loud or silently in your mind. Concentrate on God's love towards your every being. Ask God to clean not only your heart, but your mind, your soul and your entire being. You must create the purest atmosphere to get positive reception of God's intuition and that small voice that speaks directly into your heart.

Nahum 1:7

"The Lord is good, a refuge in times of trouble. He cares for those who trust in him."

3. Study God's word within the Old and New Testaments, asking God for the wisdom to discern the Bible's lessons. The parables are not easily understood the first time they are read, so you must ask for God's help in deciphering them. Only then may you apply them to your personal and professional life, as generations of God's children have done before you.

Mark 4:9-12

"Anyone with ears to hear should listen and understand" ... "You are permitted to understand the secret of the Kingdom of God. But I use parables for everything I say to outsiders, so that the Scriptures might be fulfilled."

Understand that things which you ask God for can come quickly or slowly depending on how ready you are to receive them. God knows that if he gives them to you when you are not ready, you will lose these gifts or become unable to cope with it. In time, if we use His words and apply them to our lives, we are sure to receive everything that we need or want and we may continue to ask for more.

4. Have faith that God will deliver. You can see how often many people gave up on asking things from God because they could not see any results coming out of their prayers. Most people have forgotten what the most important part of the prayer is. They forgot to get the most authoritative person to support and speed their request so that it was heard quickly by God. Much like in a court case where you need a proper barrister to work with you to ensure the judge will rule in your favour, it is the same with God. You need your spiritual brother Jesus Christ to help with your prayers so that the Heavenly Father may execute your request. Always ask God for your needs in Jesus' name. But remember, only God knows when the time is right for you to receive his gifts, much like a doctor who knows when to give treatment to his patient. Once you understand all of the above, you can use the Bible Keys and apply them to your personal life.

Isaiah 55:11

God says; "It is the same as my word. I send it out and it always produces fruit. It will accomplish all I want it to, and it will prosper everywhere I send it."

5. Finally, you must give thanks. After you have given your prayer request, you must thank God with all your heart. The more you thank Him, the quicker his blessings will come to you. You must now concentrate on believing one hundred percent in your heart that your request is now heard by God.

There is a final condition that you need to make it work. You must understand that if you have received God's answer to your request, you will now need to get to work on the request you made. You will not receive any kind of blessing that you have not earned, much like the old wives' tale of "help yourself first and God will help you."

Proverbs 10:4

"Lazy hands make a man poor, but diligent hands bring wealth."

Proverbs 22:29

"Be sure you know the condition of your flocks, give careful attention to your herds."

The above five conditions are absolute must-dos if you want your prayer to be answered and to succeed in having God bless you with wellbeing, happiness and success in your life.

Roman 10:11

"As the Scripture says. Anyone who trusts in Him will never be put to shame."

GRATITUDE

Giving thanks is of vital importance, but just Giving to others is also important!

How well do we know the meaning of the word "gratitude"? If you want Abundant Wealth from God, you must be able to change your attitude and behaviour towards what you have been given already.

1 Timothy 6:17

"..... Their trust should be in God, who richly gives us all we need for our enjoyment. Tell them to use their money to do good. They should be rich in good works and generous to those in need. By doing this they will be storing up their treasure as a good foundation for the future so that they may experience true life."

You already know how to trust in God for the things you have asked for. Now you need to know how to act while you are waiting for God to bestow upon you the things you desire. Even if you do not have much, you still need to appreciate what you do have, that which has sustained you until now.

You may hate your menial job or be in a boring business, but you must not condemn it. After all, it has kept you afloat until now.

The Key to this is that now you know how to turn things around. While appreciating what sustained you, from its original roots, God will bless it and turn it into a good thing.

Matthew 25:29
Jesus says; "For everyone who has will be given more, and they will have abundance. Whoever does not have, even what they have will be taken from them."

This first sentence above means that your need to be grateful for all the things you currently possess. This appreciation will make them become more important, even if right now they seem worthless to you. The second sentence does not mean that God will take your things away, only that without your appreciate of them, the few resources you have tend to be squandered.

In the physical realm, you may be in a job that you hate but are desperate to leave. You may want God to answer your prayers and to help you out of this predicament. In this instance, while you wait for God to manifest things that you have prayed for, you must learn to imitate God's spiritual realm in order to turn it into your real world.

Romans 8:24
".... But hope that is seen is no hope at all. Who hopes for what he already has? But we hope for what we do not yet have, we wait for it patiently."

If you know the mind of Jesus Christ, you will know that when He was in human form, everything was beautiful and perfect in God's eyes. Jesus was without worry and he was on Earth solely for the purpose of doing God's work. Nothing could harm or touch him because God's power was within him. When he was laid on the cross of crucifixion, it was because Jesus allowed himself to be, in order to fulfill the scriptures and be sacrificed as a lamb of God for all of us.

Therefore, you must have gratitude for Christ's gift because he paid with his life for your sins. You can be free of anxiety, stress, worry, distress and ill health because Jesus removed all those bad things from you. All hardships are of the physical realm; you can be free of these struggles by switching yourself to the spiritual realm.

When you know that God is by your side, your mind will be sharp and focused. No matter what sort of negative thoughts arise, you must not listen to them. They're trying to lure you away from God and all the good things that he has in store for you.

According to Christian teachings, two cosmic broadcast stations – the Light and the Dark – send signals to our brain. Any thought that is loud and clear, which urges you to react to a situation, without a proper plan, that is the enemy – the Dark. But if the thought is barely audible, if it is a soft voice emanating from the recesses of our mind, it is the song of the Light. If you are greeted with a sudden flash of intuition or inspiration, you can be certain it is from the spiritual realm.

The key to taking control of your life is to ignore the loud noise in your head and to take time to concentrate on the small, quiet sounds from God to guide you. When you succeed in blocking out the negative thoughts that manifest themselves as our greedy and selfish egos, the Light signal and all the good thoughts that come along with it are free to fill our minds. The best ideas can come forth at once and without hindrance, and you can see the way to wisdom.

In the Old Testament, during the time that king Ahab ruled in Israel, Ahab did not worship God. He killed all of God's prophets except one, Elijah. Elijah was afraid and asked for God's help. He went into a cave where he spent the night praying and waiting for God's instruction.

1 Kings 11:13

"Go out and stand before me on the mountain" the Lord told him. And as Elijah stood there, the Lord passed by, and a mighty windstorm hit the mountain. It was such a terrible blast that the rocks were torn loose, but the Lord was not in the wind. After the wind there was an earthquake, but the Lord was not in the earthquake. And after the earthquake there was a fire, but the Lord was not in the fire. And after the fire there was the sound of a gentle whisper. .... And the voice said "What are you (still) doing here, Elijah?"

Thus we can know that the gentle, whispering voice is from God, not the enemy.

You now have all the Abundant Wealth Keys in your hands, and can begin to apply them to all aspects of your life. You can begin to see success in all areas, from your personal and family life, to your professional and business life, and to your community as well.

Finally, remember this. If you care for other human beings like God cares for you, you will continue to receive God's blessing. You will please God if you lend Him a hand, doing charitable work for those less fortunate than you in this world that God has made for us all.